Surgery for Spine Disease and Intractable Pain

Surgery for Spine Disease and Intractable Pain

Special Issue Editor
Warren W. Boling

MDPI • Basel • Beijing • Wuhan • Barcelona • Belgrade • Manchester • Tokyo • Cluj • Tianjin

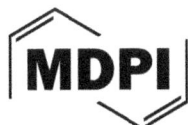

Special Issue Editor
Warren W. Boling
Department of Neurosurgery,
Loma Linda University
USA

Editorial Office
MDPI
St. Alban-Anlage 66
4052 Basel, Switzerland

This is a reprint of articles from the Special Issue published online in the open access journal *Brain Sciences* (ISSN 2076-3425) (available at: https://www.mdpi.com/journal/brainsci/special_issues/Surgery_Spine_Pain).

For citation purposes, cite each article independently as indicated on the article page online and as indicated below:

LastName, A.A.; LastName, B.B.; LastName, C.C. Article Title. *Journal Name* **Year**, *Article Number*, Page Range.

ISBN 978-3-03928-478-8 (Pbk)
ISBN 978-3-03928-479-5 (PDF)

© 2020 by the authors. Articles in this book are Open Access and distributed under the Creative Commons Attribution (CC BY) license, which allows users to download, copy and build upon published articles, as long as the author and publisher are properly credited, which ensures maximum dissemination and a wider impact of our publications.

The book as a whole is distributed by MDPI under the terms and conditions of the Creative Commons license CC BY-NC-ND.

Contents

About the Special Issue Editor vii

Warren Boling
Surgery for Spine Disease and Intractable Pain
Reprinted from: *Brain Sci.* **2020**, *10*, 62, doi:10.3390/brainsci10020062 1

Warren Boling, Minwoo Song, Wendy Shih and Bengt Karlsson
Gamma Knife Radiosurgery for Trigeminal Neuralgia: A Comparison of Dose Protocols
Reprinted from: *Brain Sci.* **2019**, *9*, 134, doi:10.3390/brainsci9060134 3

Mariagiovanna Cantone, Giuseppe Lanza, Alice Le Pira, Rita Barone, Giovanni Pennisi, Rita Bella, Manuela Pennisi and Agata Fiumara
Adjunct Diagnostic Value of Transcranial Magnetic Stimulation in Mucopolysaccharidosis-Related Cervical Myelopathy: A Pilot Study
Reprinted from: *Brain Sci.* **2019**, *9*, 200, doi:10.3390/brainsci9080200 15

Walter J. Jermakowicz, Stephanie S. Sloley, Lia Dan, Alberto Vitores, Melissa M. Carballosa-Gautam and Ian D. Hentall
Cellular Changes in Injured Rat Spinal Cord Following Electrical Brainstem Stimulation
Reprinted from: *Brain Sci.* **2019**, *9*, 124, doi:10.3390/brainsci9060124 25

Michael Hall, David Cheng, Wayne Cheng and Olumide Danisa
Antiplatelet Versus Anticoagulation for Asymptomatic Patients with Vertebral Artery Injury During Anterior Cervical Surgery—Two Case Reports and Review of Literature
Reprinted from: *Brain Sci.* **2019**, *9*, 345, doi:10.3390/brainsci9120345 37

Dinesh Ramanathan, Nikhil Sahasrabudhe and Esther Kim
Disseminated Coccidioidomycosis to the Spine—Case Series and Review of Literature
Reprinted from: *Brain Sci.* **2019**, *9*, 160, doi:10.3390/brainsci9070160 45

Wyatt McGilvery, Marc Eastin, Anish Sen and Maciej Witkos
Self Manipulated Cervical Spine Leads to Posterior Disc Herniation and Spinal Stenosis
Reprinted from: *Brain Sci.* **2019**, *9*, 125, doi:10.3390/brainsci9060125 55

Christopher Heinrich, Vadim Gospodarev, Albert Kheradpour, Craig Zuppan, Clifford C. Douglas and Tanya Minasian
Benign Giant Cell Lesion of C1 Lateral Mass: A Case Report and Literature Review
Reprinted from: *Brain Sci.* **2019**, *9*, 105, doi:10.3390/brainsci9050105 61

Gonzalo Navarro-Fernández, Lucía de-la-Puente-Ranea, Marisa Gandía-González and Alfonso Gil-Martínez
Endogenous Neurostimulation and Physiotherapy in Cluster Headache: A Clinical Case
Reprinted from: *Brain Sci.* **2019**, *9*, 60, doi:10.3390/brainsci9030060 69

About the Special Issue Editor

Warren W. Boling (Prof). Dr. Boling is Chairman of the Department of Neurosurgery at Loma Linda University and Chief of Neurosurgery at Loma Linda University Hospital. Additionally, he directs the surgery of epilepsy program at Loma Linda University. Dr. Boling has a particular interest in elevating the medical and surgical treatment of neurological diseases in underserved regions of the world.

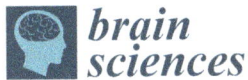

Editorial

Surgery for Spine Disease and Intractable Pain

Warren Boling

Department of Neurosurgery, Loma Linda University, Loma Linda, CA 92354, USA; WBoling@llu.edu

Received: 24 December 2019; Accepted: 19 January 2020; Published: 24 January 2020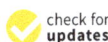

Painful conditions, particularly due to head pain, spinal disease, and neuropathic pain, are highly prevalent in modern society, resulting in a significant impact on the individual due to the disability of the condition and the direct cost of associated treatments. Additionally, indirect costs to society result from the loss of work productivity of the individual due to pain. For musculoskeletal pain alone, the related costs in the USA are estimated at $215 billion, of which 41% are from direct medical care, and the remaining are indirect costs associated with the condition [1]. The impact on society of head pain is manifest by the fact that this chief complaint is the fifth leading cause of visits to the Emergency Department and an even more common chief complaint for women aged 15–64 years [2].

In this Special Issue of Brain Sciences, the included manuscripts have explored several causes of pain and disability, their diagnosis, and treatment. Cantone et al. evaluated the disability that can result from mucopolysaccharidosis related cervical myelopathy [3]. The authors found that motor evoked potential measured from transcranial magnetic stimulation is a promising diagnostic tool to evaluate for early myelopathy before symptoms become overt. Trigeminal neuralgia is a severe and disabling face pain that can be effectively treated surgically in most people when medicines fail. Boling et al. reported their experience with different radiosurgery dosing protocols to target the root entry zone of the trigeminal nerve in the treatment of medically intractable trigeminal neuralgia [4]. The authors found that a higher dose regimen of 85Gy was the most effective and durable treatment for the facial pain. Spinal cord injury is an important cause of disability due to paralysis and loss of function as well as frequently associated neuropathic pain. Jermakowicz et al. evaluated the mechanisms underlying low-frequency electrical stimulation and the ability of stimulation to improve motor recovery and lessen allodynia related to spinal cord injury [5]. In the experiments performed, rats received a spinal cord injury at the cervical spinal level. The authors then identified that low-frequency electrical stimulation of the animals' hindbrain nucleus raphe magnus resulted in decreased counts of cells related to neuro-inflammation and an increase in radial glia, which serve as a scaffold for neuronal migration in the area of injury. The findings of this study suggest a potential role for neuromodulatory therapies in the management of spinal cord injury and its sequelae. Hall et al. described an iatrogenic injury related to the treatment of a painful spine condition, then reviewed the literature of the treatment options available [6]. Vertebral artery injury is a rare but potentially devastating complication of surgery of the cervical spine. Surgery of the cervical spine is most commonly performed for pain related to instability, arthritic degenerative disease, or radicular pain resulting from nerve root compression. The authors reviewed treatment options and concluded that antiplatelet or anticoagulation were both options for the treatment of iatrogenic vertebral artery injury, and neither medical management approach has been found to be superior. Coccidioidomycosis is a fungal infectious disease caused by the Coccidioides species endemic to the Southwestern United States. Although this disease is rare, in endemic regions, Coccidioidomycosis can spread to the bone and spine, resulting in a destructive spinal disease. Ramanathan et al. described their institutions experience with spinal Coccidioidomycosis and reviewed the modern treatment approaches to this potentially devastating disease [7]. McGilvery et al. presented an unusual case of acute cervical disc herniation causing neurological deficit that resulted from self-manipulation of the cervical spine [8]. Heinrich et al. described a rare case of a primary osseous tumor of the spinal column of a 15 year old patient that required surgical decompression [9]. The authors described the surgical approach to a destructive lesion in C1 and the histopathology and radiology of a benign giant cell tumor of the spine. Chronic cluster headaches are a disabling form of headache characterized by severe unilateral pain in short-duration episodes, which are associated with ipsilateral autonomic symptoms primarily involving the temporal, supraorbital, and infraorbital head areas. Navarro-Fernández et al. described the value of a multimodal approach to treat this severe form of headache, which can include pharmacology, neurostimulation, and physiotherapy [10]. The authors presented a patient from their clinic who benefitted from a novel treatment combination of occipital nerve neurostimulation and physiotherapy approaches for chronic cluster headache. The authors went on to describe a mechanistic hypothesis for the headache resolution resulting from the different modes of treatment. The enormity of the topic of spine disease, pain, and disability could never be adequately covered in a single publication. However, this Special Issue provides valuable insights into a few of the most disabling pain conditions that affect mankind.

Conflicts of Interest: The authors declare no conflicts of interest.

References

1. Baldwin, M.L. Reducing the costs of work-related musculoskeletal disorders: Targeting strategies to chronic disability cases. *J. Electromyogr. Kinesiol.* **2004**, *14*, 33–41. [CrossRef] [PubMed]
2. Smitherman, T.A.; Burch, R.; Sheikh, H.; Loder, E. The prevalence, impact, and treatment of migraine and severe headaches in the United States: A review of statistics from national surveillance studies. *Headache* **2013**, *53*, 427–436. [CrossRef] [PubMed]
3. Cantone, M.; Lanza, G.; Le Pira, A.; Barone, R.; Pennisi, G.; Bella, R.; Pennisi, M.; Fiumara, A. Adjunct Diagnostic Value of Transcranial Magnetic Stimulation in Mucopolysaccharidosis-Related Cervical Myelopathy: A Pilot Study. *Brain Sci.* **2019**, *9*, 200. [CrossRef] [PubMed]
4. Boling, W.; Song, M.; Shih, W.; Karlsson, B. Gamma Knife Radiosurgery for Trigeminal Neuralgia: A Comparison of Dose Protocols. *Brain Sci.* **2019**, *9*, 134. [CrossRef] [PubMed]
5. Jermakowicz, W.J.; Sloley, S.S.; Dan, L.; Vitores, A.; Carballosa-Gautam, M.M.; Hentall, I.D. Cellular Changes in Injured Rat Spinal Cord Following Electrical Brainstem Stimulation. *Brain Sci.* **2019**, *9*, 124. [CrossRef] [PubMed]
6. Hall, M.; Cheng, D.; Cheng, W.; Danisa, O. Antiplatelet Versus Anticoagulation for Asymptomatic Patients with Vertebral Artery Injury During Anterior Cervical Surgery—Two Case Reports and Review of Literature. *Brain Sci.* **2019**, *9*, 345. [CrossRef] [PubMed]
7. Ramanathan, D.; Sahasrabudhe, N.; Kim, E. Disseminated Coccidioidomycosis to the Spine—Case Series and Review of Literature. *Brain Sci.* **2019**, *9*, 160. [CrossRef] [PubMed]
8. McGilvery, W.; Eastin, M.; Sen, A.; Witkos, M. Self Manipulated Cervical Spine Leads to Posterior Disc Herniation and Spinal Stenosis. *Brain Sci.* **2019**, *9*, 125. [CrossRef] [PubMed]
9. Heinrich, C.; Gospodarev, V.; Kheradpour, A.; Zuppan, C.; Douglas, C.C.; Minasian, T. Benign Giant Cell Lesion of C1 Lateral Mass: A Case Report and Literature Review. *Brain Sci.* **2019**, *9*, 105. [CrossRef] [PubMed]
10. Navarro-Fernández, G.; de-la-Puente-Ranea, L.; Gandía-González, M.; Gil-Martínez, A. Endogenous Neurostimulation and Physiotherapy in Cluster Headache: A Clinical Case. *Brain Sci.* **2019**, *9*, 60.

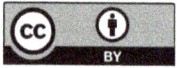

© 2020 by the author. Licensee MDPI, Basel, Switzerland. This article is an open access article distributed under the terms and conditions of the Creative Commons Attribution (CC BY) license (http://creativecommons.org/licenses/by/4.0/).

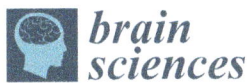

Article

Gamma Knife Radiosurgery for Trigeminal Neuralgia: A Comparison of Dose Protocols

Warren Boling [1,*], Minwoo Song [1], Wendy Shih [2] and Bengt Karlsson [3]

1 Department of Neurosurgery, Loma Linda University, Loma Linda, CA 92354, USA; MINSong@llu.edu
2 School of Public Health, Loma Linda University, Loma Linda, CA 92354, USA; wshih@llu.edu
3 Department of Neurosurgery, National University Hospital, Singapore 119228, Singapore; nykuttram@yahoo.se
* Correspondence: wboling@LLU.edu; Tel.: +1-(909)-558-4419; Fax: +1-(909)-558-4825

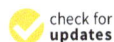

Received: 24 April 2019; Accepted: 4 June 2019; Published: 10 June 2019

Abstract: Purpose: A variety of treatment plans including an array of prescription doses have been used in radiosurgery treatment of trigeminal neuralgia (TN). However, despite a considerable experience in the radiosurgical treatment of TN, an ideal prescription dose that balances facial dysesthesia risk with pain relief durability has not been determined. Methods and Materials: This retrospective study of patients treated with radiosurgery for typical TN evaluates two treatment doses in relation to outcomes of pain freedom, bothersome facial numbness, and patient satisfaction with treatment. All patients were treated with radiosurgery for intractable and disabling TN. A treatment dose protocol change from 80 to 85 Gy provided an opportunity to compare two prescription doses. The variables evaluated were pain relief, treatment side-effect profile, and patient satisfaction. Results: Typical TN was treated with 80 Gy in 26 patients, and 85 Gy in 37 patients. A new face sensory disturbance was reported after 80 Gy in 16% and after 85 Gy in 27% ($p = 0.4$). Thirteen failed an 80 Gy dose whereas seven failed an 85 Gy dose. Kaplan–Meier analysis found that at 29 months 50% failed an 80 Gy treatment compared with 79% who had durable pain relief after 85 Gy treatment ($p = 0.04$). Conclusion: The 85 Gy dose for TN provided a more durable pain relief compared to the 80 Gy one without a significantly elevated occurrence of facial sensory disturbance.

Keywords: trigeminal neuralgia; tic douloureux; radiosurgery; Gamma Knife

1. Introduction

Trigeminal neuralgia (TN) is a chronic neuropathic pain condition that affects the regions of the face innervated by the trigeminal nerve. Typical TN causes severe and sudden volleys of shock-like facial pain that lasts a few seconds to a few minutes in the distribution of one or more divisions of the trigeminal nerve. When patients experience attacks of pain that come on repeatedly, the result is a pain condition that is disabling in nature. Typical TN will have a trigger in the trigeminal nerve division distribution the pain is felt in, which often leads to aversive behavior by the patient to avoid the pain. For example, a trigger inside the mouth may make eating so difficult that poor nutrition results.

Atypical forms of face pain have symptoms that are not shock-like in nature, do not follow the trigeminal nerve distribution, and/or do not have an associated trigger. Atypical face pain my certainly be disabling in nature, however, the treatment options available to typical TN patients are less likely to benefit individuals with atypical face pain.

The etiology of typical TN in most cases is due to vascular compression at the nerve root entry zone as the trigeminal nerve exits the pons. In these cases, microvascular decompression surgery (MVD) in which a small sponge is placed as a cushion between the trigeminal nerve and the offending vessel has a high success rate in eliminating the TN pain. However, the associated risks and inconvenience related to the open surgical procedure of MVD lead many individuals with disabling pain, in particular more elderly and frail individuals, to seek out less-invasive treatment approaches such as radiosurgery and percutaneous rhizotomy. Both these approaches have a good success rate in eliminating the pain of TN, but pain recurrence is generally more common compared with MVD.

Lars Leksell introduced radiosurgery as a treatment of trigeminal neuralgia (TN) at the Karolinska Institute in the 1950s [1]. Although interest waned in treating TN with radiosurgery until the early 1990s when there was a substantial increase in the published literature concerning radiosurgery for TN. There is now over the past couple of decades considerable patient experience with radiosurgery in the treatment of TN with the vast majority of publications demonstrating benefit for the severe disabling facial pain [2], particularly in the elderly population who make up the majority of individuals with TN treated by radiosurgery [3].

Radiosurgery treatment variables that have potential to impact both long-term pain relief and occurrence of treatment side-effects include the radiation dose delivered to the nerve, volume or extent of the nerve treated, and anatomical localization of the treatment target. Of these variables, treatment dose has been most frequently studied. Yet, despite a substantial experience in the radiosurgery community, the optimum radiosurgery prescription dose for TN has not been determined.

Herein, the authors present results from their patients with medically intractable TN treated using Gamma Knife radiosurgery (GKR). A retrospective comparison of two treatment dose plans of 80 and 85 Gy was analyzed for the treatment of typical TN. The variables assessed were pain relief, side-effect profile, and patient satisfaction.

2. Material and Methods

2.1. Patient Population

All patients were treated for medically intractable TN by the authors at a single institution over a seven year period. Patients (or a family member if the patient was deceased or unable to provide answers to a questionnaire) were contacted by phone or had a face-to-face interview to compete a study questionnaire at follow-up time points after treatment had been completed. The questionnaire inquired about timing of pain relief after GKR, quality and severity of pain, and side effects or complications related to GKR. The patient's subjective assessment of GKR and treatment satisfaction was evaluated by asking two questions: "Are you pleased with GKR?" and "Would you have the procedure again?".

2.2. GKR Treatment Plan

Gamma Knife Model 4c (Elekta, Stockholm, Sweden) was used for all treatments. The treatment plan centered the maximum dose on the root entry zone (REZ) of the proximal trigeminal nerve with the 30% isodose line just contacting the brainstem. Treatment was performed using a 4 mm collimated single shot. The earlier treatment plan was with a prescription maximum dose delivered to patients of 80 Gy. Later, the protocol was changed to a prescription maximum dose of 85 Gy in all subsequent patients. These two dose plans were analyzed and compared in treated patients for variables of pain relief, facial numbness, complications of treatment, and patient satisfaction (Figure 1).

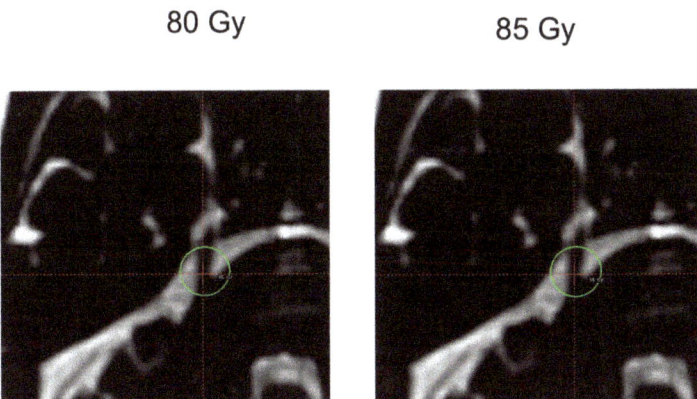

Figure 1. Images of typical corresponding dose plans with the maximum dose targeting the root entry zone (REZ). Green circle is the 15 Gy isodose line.

2.3. Statistics

A Kaplan–Meier statistic analyzed the duration of pain freedom after GKR for low- and high-dose groups of patients. The Kaplan–Meier (K–M) survival distributions of the two dose groups were compared using the log rank test. A Fisher's exact or chi square test compared categorical data, such as new onset facial numbness after GKR, patient satisfaction queries, and Barrow Neurological Institute pain intensity (BNI) at last follow-up [4]. $p < 0.05$ was considered significant.

3. Results

A total of 68 patients were treated with GKR for intractable TN over seven years. Three patients with multiple sclerosis (MS) (all in the 80 Gy group), and two with no available follow-up after treatment (one in each group) were excluded from the analysis. Therefore, in patients with typical TN and post-treatment follow-up, the treatment dose was 80 Gy in 26 individuals, and 85 Gy was delivered to 37 individuals. Mean patient age was 71 years. Twenty-seven were women. Fifteen patients had a procedure for TN prior to GKR (10 in the 80 Gy group, $p = 0.6$). The mean follow-up after GKR in pain free patients was 37 months (range 6–72 months) in individuals treated with 80 Gy and 26 months (range 6–52 months) in patients treated with 85 Gy.

A new facial sensory disturbance was reported after an 80 Gy treatment dose in four patients (16%) and in 10 (27%) after an 85 Gy treatment dose ($p = 0.4$). Only one individual reported being bothered by numbness in the 80 Gy group and two reported that the sensory change was bothersome in the 85 Gy group. Patients answered "No" to either question of treatment satisfaction (Are you pleased with GKR? or Would you have the procedure again?) in 22% of the 85 Gy treatment group and in 44% of the 80 Gy treatment group ($p = 0.09$).

BNI pain scores at last follow-up were evaluated in each patient. Pain freedom without medication (BNI score of I) was realized in eight individuals treated with 80 Gy and in 21 treated with 85 Gy, which represented more pain freedom without medication in the 85 Gy group ($p = 0.04$). In addition, significantly more patients who received 85 Gy treatment experienced an overall good result (BNI score I, II, and III) than patients treated with 80 Gy (29 with overall good results in the 85 Gy group versus 14 in the 80 Gy group, $p = 0.04$).

A survival curve was analyzed for both treatment groups using the Kaplan–Meier statistic (K–M). Recurrent severe pain despite medication or persisting severe pain after GKR was deemed a treatment failure. At the last follow-up, thirteen patients (52%) who received 80 Gy treatment dose failed GKR whereas seven patients (19%) failed GKR after 85 Gy. K–M analysis found at the 29 months time point that 50% of patients had failed 80 Gy GKR treatment, and at the same time point, 79% of patients had continued pain relief after receiving 85 GY treatment (Figure 2). The K–M analysis demonstrated a significant difference in the achievement of pain relief and durability of response at 29 months ($p = 0.04$).

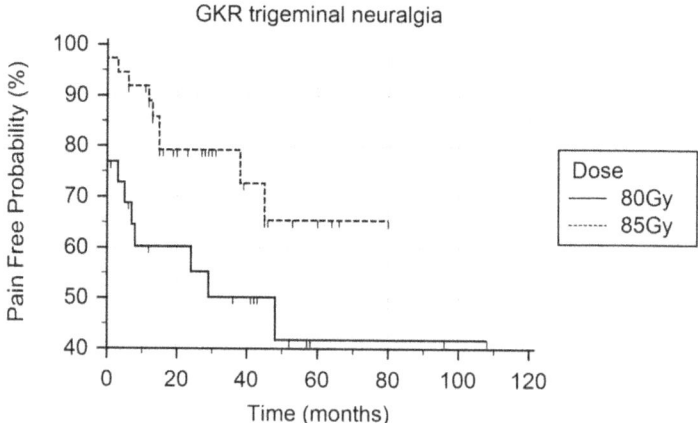

Figure 2. Kaplan–Meier analysis of Gamma Knife radiosurgery for trigeminal neuralgia using two treatment doses. Log rank test demonstrated improved durability and more patients with pain relief in the 85 Gy treated group ($p = 0.04$).

Potential confounders of treatment success were evaluated to determine whether age, new numbness after GKR, surgery before GKR, or length of follow-up differed by GKR dosage (Figure 3). There were significant differences in age and prior surgery in the two GKR dosage groups. As a separate analysis, the effect of dosage on becoming pain free was analyzed while adjusting for potential confounders. In addition, only the effect of age and prior surgery were evaluated as possible confounders. For both analyses, the confounders were found to be not significantly contributing to the dose effect on pain freedom.

	80 Gy	85 Gy	*p*-Value
Age (years)	67.77 (13.57)	74.1 (9.78)	0.04
Length of Follow-up	41.3 (26.01)	30.26 (21.60)	0.07
New Numbness after GKR			0.07
No	27 (90%)	27 (71%)	
Yes	3 (10%)	11 (29%)	
Surgery Prior to GKR			0.002
No	16 (53%)	33 (89%)	
Yes	14 (47%)	4 (11%)	

Figure 3. Analysis of potential confounders to pain freedom in the two dosage groups. Patient age and a procedure for trigeminal neuralgia prior to Gamma Knife radiosurgery (GKR) were both found to be significantly different between the dosage groups.

4. Discussion

Kondziolka et al. identified that patients who received a 70 Gy dose for treatment of TN fared better with improved pain relief compared to lower prescription doses, and complications were rare [5]. Also, the authors suggested in their patient population that higher treatment doses over 70 Gy yielded even better TN pain relief. However, unresolved is the ideal dose that provides the best-possible pain control balanced with the minimum associated radiation complications (Table 1). Additionally, there is no agreement in the published reports of dose escalation. Some authors have identified no benefit for TN or absence of improved pain relief from treatment with higher prescription doses ranging between 50 and 90 Gy [6–12]. For example, although an improvement in absolute pain relief was not found by Kim et al. with a higher radiation dose, these authors reported 85 Gy provided a more rapid response of pain relief after radiosurgery compared with the 80 Gy dose [13]. Consistent with our results, other authors have identified definite improved pain relief with dose escalation [14–18]. Longhi et al. evaluated radiosurgery for TN targeting the trigeminal nerve root entry zone. The authors identified higher doses in the 80–90 Gy range to be the most effective radiosurgery dose related to a pain free outcome that additionally had low risk of sensory disturbance, although this risk was elevated with the highest treatment dose [14].

Table 1. Studies of prescription dose comparison in radiosurgery of trigeminal neuralgia. * Linear accelerator radiosurgery, REZ = dorsal root entry zone, RG = retrogasserian.

Study	Max Dose to Nerve	Dose Related Pain Freedom	Facial Numbness Dose Related	Radiosurgery Target
Kondziolka et al. [5]	≤65 Gy ≥70 Gy	Yes ≥ 70 Gy $p = 0.02$	No relationship	REZ
Pollock et al. [8]	70 Gy 90 Gy	No difference	Yes. Numbness and dysesthesia	REZ
Alpert et al. [14]	≤80 Gy 85 Gy ≥90 Gy	Yes, with escalating doses $p < 0.001$	No relationship	REZ ±second shot 3–4 mm more distal
Sheehan et al. [9]	50–90 Gy	No difference	No relationship	REZ
Tawk et al. [10]	70, 80, or 90 Gy	No difference	Trend to dose relationship	REZ
Morbidini-Gaffney et al. [18]	<80 Gy 85 Gy >85 Gy	Yes < 85 Gy $p < 0.001$		REZ ±second shot 2–4 mm more distal
Régis et al. [11]	70–90 Gy	No difference	No relationship	7.5 mm anterior to pons
Fountas et al. [7]	75–85 Gy	No difference		REZ
Longhi et al. [15]	75–95 Gy >80 Gy	Yes > 80 Gy $p = 0.008$	>90 Gy increased numbness	REZ
Chen et al. * [6]	85 or 90 Gy	No difference		Cisternal nerve segment
Matsuda et al. [16]	80 or 90 Gy	No difference	Trend to more numbness in 90 Gy RG target	80 Gy REZ 90 Gy RG target
Kim et al. [13]	75 or 85 Gy	No difference	No relationship	REZ
Smith et al. * [17]	70 or 90 Gy	Yes, at one year	Trend to dose relationship	REZ
Zhang et al. [12]	75 or 90 Gy	No difference	No dose relationship	Cisternal portion of nerve with one or two isocenters
Kotecha et al. [19]	≤82, 83–86, or ≥90 Gy	Improved > 82 Gy	No dose relationship prescription doses ≥ 83 Gy	REZ
Massager et al. [20]	70–85 Gy, 90 Gy, or 90 Gy with shielding	No, trend to better pain freedom in higher dose	Yes. Numbness related with higher dose	Anterior cisternal nerve segment
Villavicencio et al. * [21]	Range of 50–80 Gy, median 75 Gy	Yes, related with longer nerve segment treated	Yes	REZ

Morbidini-Gaffney et al., in a follow-on study of patients reported in Alpert et al. [14], assessed patients treated with TN in order to evaluate efficacy of two versus one-isocenter treatment plans as well as an evaluation of radiation dose escalation [18]. The results were that two isocenters plus patients receiving greater than 85 Gy had a longer duration of good treatment response compared with lower treatment doses and a single isocenter. There were no identified facial dysesthesias although

11% reported mild facial numbness. In a conflicting report from Zhang et al. patients with refractory TN were treated with a maximum dose of 75–90 Gy using either one ($n = 41$) or two ($n = 32$) isocenters. The authors found no difference in pain relief or sensory disturbance with higher dose, but the patients with multiple-isocenter treatment plans did experience more numbness or paresthesia in the trigeminal distribution [12].

Smith et al. used linear accelerator-based radiosurgery to treat TN [17]. Over an initial time period, 28 patients received doses between 70 and 85 Gy. The subsequently treated 82 patients were prescribed a radiation dose of 90 Gy, with a treatment plan of the 30% isodose line touching the brainstem. The treatment plan was further modified later with the goal of increasing the dose at the root entry zone so that the 50% isodose line was tangential to the pons in 59 patients. Patients treated with 90 Gy had superior pain relief at one year follow-up and more rapid resolution of pain relief after treatment. There was no significant difference in facial numbness between the treatment groups. Young et al. reported over a five year follow-up after 90 Gy GKR treatment for TN that over 70% of patients were pain free with or without medication [22]. The authors concluded that higher-dose treatment was effective in treating TN, that pain relief was more likely in patients with facial numbness post treatment, and the authors commented that a 90 Gy prescription dose may be associated with an increase in bothersome sensory complications in comparison with lower treatment doses. Pollock et al. also identified increased numbness and dysesthesia in their patients treated with 90 Gy compared with lower doses [23]. The University of CaliforniaSan Diego TN treatment experience was reviewed by Taich et al., who identified elevated risk of bothersome facial numbness with treatment doses greater than 85 Gy [24]. Radiosurgery dose escalation was studied retrospectively in 870 TN patients by Kotecha et al. who analyzed patients divided into groups of delivered doses: ≤82, 83–86, and ≥90 Gy [19]. The investigators identified that dose escalation above 82 Gy resulted in improved pain relief, but with elevated risk of treatment-related facial numbness. However, facial numbness resulted in similar proportions in patients treated at prescription doses ≥83 Gy. Massager et al. [20] analyzed 358 patients with GKR-treated TN that targeted the anterior cisternal portion of the trigeminal nerve. The Brussels study divided patients into three different dosimetric treatment groups, which revealed rates of trigeminal numbness and pain relief closely related to the radiation dose delivered to the retrogasserian portion of the nerve. A similar relationship was reported by Villavicencio et al. [21]. This group treated TN using CyberKnife (Accuray Inc., Sunnyvale, CA, USA) radiosurgery, which resulted in better pain relief and increased hypesthesia rates in those patients receiving higher radiation dose with a longer nerve segment treated.

High-resolution MRI or CT myelography allows for the trigeminal nerve to be clearly delineated from its exit at the brainstem to Meckel's cave. The imaging well-defined anatomy of the trigeminal nerve allows for accurate radiosurgery targeting at any point along its course in the subarachnoid cistern. The REZ has been the most common radiosurgery treatment site of TN likely because the REZ has a long history in neurosurgery as a lesioning target for a variety of pain conditions. However, in an effort to reduce the pontine radiation dose, some radiosurgery users have moved the target more anteriorly along the nerve [17]; although, few investigators have critically analyzed anatomical targeting differences related to outcome from treatment of TN (Table 2). Among the few authors who have critically evaluated a more anterior treatment plan, Matsuda et al. found no difference in pain freedom and a trend to more facial numbness using an anterior retrogasserian target in comparison to a REZ target, although the anterior target received a higher dose in their patients [16]. Park et al. identified no difference in pain freedom or facial numbness in patients treated with REZ versus an anterior retrogasserian target [25]. Rashid et al. treated with 90 Gy maximum dose to REZ and retrogasserian targets. Comparison of the two treatment groups identified improved pain freedom in the REZ target patients, and no difference in the development of new facial numbness [26]. Xu et al. retrospectively evaluated 141 patients with TN treated using GKR prescribed to a maximum dose of 80 Gy targeting either the REZ or the retrogasserian nerve. Their analysis revealed the REZ provided more durable pain relief with similar initial efficacy, but that facial numbness was more common in the

REZ-treated patients [27]. Sharim et al., using linear accelerator-based radiosurgery, found no benefit in regard to face hypesthesia and no difference in pain relief rate with trigeminal nerve targets more anterior to the REZ [28]. Strategies such as anterior nerve targeting as well as techniques to correct dosimetry are effective in reduction of the brainstem total dose [29], and there is limited evidence that the risk of facial numbness may be reduced with a more anterior treatment target. This topic was reviewed by the International Radiosurgery Society Practice Guideline committee, which concluded that there is level II evidence that an anterior target reduces radiosurgery-related facial numbness with a similar benefit of pain reduction compared to REZ [30].

Table 2. Comparison studies of radiosurgery targets in the treatment of trigeminal neuralgia (TN). REZ = dorsal root entry zone.

Study	Radiosurgery Target and Max Dose to Nerve	Pain Freedom	Facial Numbness Target Related
Matsuda et al. [16]	80 Gy REZ 90 Gy retrogasserian target	No difference	Trend to more numbness in the anterior target patients
Park et al. [25]	80–90 Gy REZ or retrogasserian target	No difference	No relationship
Xu et al. [27]	80 Gy REZ or retrogasserian target	Similar initial pain relief. REZ more durable	More facial numbness in the REZ target patients
Rashid et al. [26]	90 Gy REZ or retrogasserian target	REZ target better pain control	No relationship

A few reports have described treating a greater nerve volume in an effort to improve pain-free results by employing an additional isocenter along the length of the nerve (Table 3). In a prospective randomized study, Flickinger et al. found an elevated risk of facial numbness with a two-isocenter treatment plan without improved pain relief [31]. However, in other published studies, Pollock et al. [8] and Alpert et al. [14] identified no relationship between nerve volume treatment and the development of facial numbness. Morbidini-Gaffney et al. [18], in a follow-on study from Alpert et al. [14], described in their patient population a significant positive correlation of multiple isocenters and higher treatment dose with pain freedom. They reported mild numbness in 11% of patients, although the hypesthesia risk associated with different treatment plans was not clear in the publication. Zhao et al. reported 247 patients who underwent a multi-isocenter GKR treatment of two adjacent 4 mm shots distributed along the trigeminal nerve with a maximum dose of 88 Gy [32]. In this group of patients treated, facial numbness occurred in 32.0%, of which 3.6% were identified as bothersome. Wolf et al. found in their TN patents treated with GKR no relationship of pain freedom with nerve length or nerve volume treated [33]. The authors did identify a relationship of better durability of pain relief at one year in patients with higher treatment dose delivered to smaller nerve volumes. Overall new facial numbness was reported in 23.6%, although only 3.6% experienced bothersome numbness. The preponderance of published studies analyzing multiple-isocenter treatment plans found no difference in pain-free outcome from more than one treatment shot, and that treatment-related facial numbness is not a consistently identified relationship with multi-shot treatment plans. However, the best evidence to date was from a single prospective randomized study [31], which found a significantly elevated risk of sensory changes related with a two-isocenter plan.

Hypesthesia was rare in our patients (22% of all individuals treated for TN) with no difference between the two treatment doses. Most individuals treated by the authors who developed a sensory disturbance were not bothered by the numbness, typically patients commented that an improved quality of life resulting from resolution of the disabling pain was more relevant compared to the sensory change. Some patients also commented that a new facial numbness was an acceptable trade-off for pain relief. However, it should be noted that in three patients (21% of patients with a post-treatment sensory disturbance and 5% of all treated patients) bothersome sensory change was GKR treatment related, and the resulting dysesthesia in these individuals is reasonably regarded as a toxicity of the radiosurgery treatment. Seventy-eight percent of patients treated with 85 Gy maximum dose to the trigeminal nerve responded that they were pleased with the GKR and would choose the treatment again, which is similar to other reports of patient satisfaction. Debono et al. reported 86.5% patient satisfaction with LINAC radiosurgery of 90 Gy dose for trigeminal neuralgia [34].

Table 3. Radiosurgery studies of multi-isocenter treatment plans. REZ = dorsal root entry zone.

Study	Max Dose to Nerve	Pain Freedom	Facial Numbness	Radiosurgery Target
Flickinger et al. [31]	75 Gy one or two isocenters	No difference	Increased numbness with two isocenters	REZ ±second shot 2–4 mm distal to brainstem
Pollock et al. [23]	70–90 Gy one or two isocenters	Trend for longer length of treated nerve	No relation with nerve volume treated	Single anterior target ±second shot along nerve
Alpert et al. [14]	≤80, 85, or ≥90 Gy one or two isocenters	Improved with escalating dose, two-shot treatment received higher dose	No relation with nerve volume treated	REZ ±second shot 3–4 mm more distal
Morbidini-Gaffney et al. [18]	<80, 85, or >85 Gy one or two isocenters	Improved in ≥85 Gy dose and number of isocenters treated	11% mild numbness, unknown relation to number of isocenters	REZ ±second shot 2–4 mm more distal
Zhang et al. Neurol India, [12]	75–90 Gy, one or two isocenters	No difference detected in dose delivered or number of isocenters	Numbness or paresthesia increased with two isocenter treatment	Cisternal portion of trigeminal nerve
Zhao et al. [32]	88 Gy and two isocenters		32% numbness 3.6% bothersome numbness	Two adjacent 4 mm shots commencing at the REZ
Wolf et al. [33]	80–90 Gy initial GKR, 65–70 Gy repeat GKR, 80 Gy shorter-nerve treatment, 85 Gy longer-nerve treatment	No relationship to nerve length or volume treated More durable in higher dose to smaller volume	Numbness in 23.6%, bothersome in 3.6%	REZ

Interventions that impact neural function are typically described as either ablative or modulatory. This has been discussed by other authors in regard to treatment of TN [35,36]. A seeming contradiction in discussions of radiosurgery for TN is that facial numbness resulting from radiosurgery is commonly labeled a treatment complication. A degree of facial numbness in the trigeminal branch of pain is a desired result of an ablative technique such as radiofrequency lesioning, which correlates positively with pain relief [37]. In fact, radiosurgery is more likely to yield pain relief in patients experiencing a facial sensory deficit, a fact that argues for an ablative mechanism [22,38]. However, neuromodulation is a better description of radiosurgery in the majority of patients who are able to realize pain relief without a sensory disturbance. Likewise, a dose–response relationship with hypesthesia has not been clearly demonstrated in studies of dose escalation (Table 1). In animal models of radiosurgery, a histopathological dose relationship has been demonstrated [39,40]. Minor changes become evident at about 80 Gy and necrosis is seen after the delivery of 100 Gy to the trigeminal nerve. In general, investigations up to now support elements of both neuromodulation and ablation as the physiological mechanism underlying radiosurgery treatment of TN, particularly at the radiation doses used to treat patients.

The optimal radiosurgery treatment dose for TN should strike a balance between providing the most robust pain relief and the least possible risk of radiation-induced complications. The only radiation-related complication identified in our patient population was hemifacial dysesthesia, which was rare (4% in the 80 Gy treatment group and 5.4% in the 85 Gy group) and not significantly different between the two prescription doses. However, the patients who received the higher treatment dose of 85 Gy did realize a more robust treatment response compared with those who received the 80 Gy dose (79% versus 50% pain relief, respectively, at 29 months, K–M analysis, $p = 0.04$). The major limitations of our study are a retrospective analysis of outcome measures and a shorter follow-up period in the high-dose, 85 Gy, treatment group.

5. Conclusions

We identified in our patients with typical TN that a GKR prescription dose treatment of 85 Gy provided a longer lasting and more robust pain relief compared to a dose of 80 Gy. A facial sensory change occurred in 11% more of the individuals in the 85 Gy treatment group, although the difference did not reach statistical significance ($p = 0.4$). Dysesthesia or a bothersome facial numbness was rare, and these complications were equally distributed between the treatment groups. The majority of patients were satisfied with radiosurgery for TN and, as expected, patients treated with the more effective dose of 85 Gy demonstrated a trend of greater treatment satisfaction. However, there is no agreement in the published studies of efficacy of dose escalation for the radiosurgical treatment of TN, and determination of the ideal dose prescription that maximizes pain relief and minimizes dysesthesia will likely require a randomized prospective clinical trial.

Author Contributions: All authors contributed substantially and meaningfully to the manuscript and research: Conceptualization, W.B. and B.K.; methodology, W.B.; investigation, W.B.; data curation, W.B. and B.K.; writing—review and editing, W.B., M.S., and B.K.

Conflicts of Interest: The authors declare no conflict of interest.

References

1. Niranjan, A.; Maitz, A.H.; Lunsford, A.; Gerszten, P.C.; Flickinger, J.C.; Kondziolka, D.; Lunsford, L.D. Radiosurgery techniques and current devices. *Prog. Neurol. Surg.* **2007**, *20*, 50–67. [PubMed]
2. Régis, J.; Tuleasca, C. Fifteen years of Gamma Knife surgery for trigeminal neuralgia in the Journal of Neurosurgery. History of a revolution in functional neurosurgery. *J. Neurosurg.* **2011**, *115*, 2–7. [CrossRef] [PubMed]
3. Cohen, J.; Mousavi, S.H.; Faraji, A.H.; Akpinar, B.; Monaco, E.A.; Flickinger, J.C.; Niranjan, A.; Lunsford, L.D. Stereotactic Radiosurgery as Initial Surgical Management for Elderly Patients with Trigeminal Neuralgia. *Stereotact. Funct. Neurosurg.* **2017**, *95*, 158–165. [CrossRef] [PubMed]
4. Rogers, C.L.; Shetter, A.G.; Fiedler, J.A.; Smith, K.A.; Han, P.P.; Speiser, B.L. Gamma knife radiosurgery for trigeminal neuralgia: the initial experience of The Barrow Neurological Institute. *Int. J. Radiat. Oncol. Biol. Phys.* **2000**, *47*, 1013–1019. [CrossRef]
5. Kondziolka, D.; Lunsford, L.D.; Flickinger, J.C.; Young, R.F.; Vermeulen, S.; Duma, C.M.; Jacques, D.B.; Rand, R.W.; Regis, J.; Peragut, J.C.; et al. Stereotactic radiosurgery for trigeminal neuralgia: A multiinstitutional study using the gamma unit. *J. Neurosurg.* **1996**, *84*, 940–945. [CrossRef] [PubMed]
6. Chen, J.C.; Greathouse, H.E.; Girvigian, M.R.; Miller, M.J.; Liu, A.; Rahimian, J. Prognostic factors for radiosurgery treatment of trigeminal neuralgia. *Neurosurgery* **2008**, *62*, A53–A60. [CrossRef] [PubMed]
7. Fountas, K.N.; Smith, J.R.; Lee, G.P.; Jenkins, P.D.; Cantrell, R.R.; Sheils, W.C. Gamma Knife stereotactic radiosurgical treatment of idiopathic trigeminal neuralgia: Long-term outcome and complications. *Neurosurg. Focus* **2007**, *23*, E8. [CrossRef] [PubMed]
8. Pollock, B.E.; Phuong, L.K.; Foote, R.L.; Stafford, S.L.; Gorman, D.A. High-dose trigeminal neuralgia radiosurgery associated with increased risk of trigeminal nerve dysfunction. *Neurosurgery* **2001**, *49*, 58–62. [PubMed]
9. Sheehan, J.; Pan, H.C.; Stroila, M.; Steiner, L. Gamma knife surgery for trigeminal neuralgia: Outcomes and prognostic factors. *J. Neurosurg.* **2005**, *102*, 434–441. [CrossRef] [PubMed]
10. Tawk, R.G.; Duffy-Fronckowiak, M.; Scott, B.E.; Alberico, R.A.; Diaz, A.Z.; Podgorsak, M.B.; Plunkett, R.J.; Fenstermaker, R.A. Stereotactic gamma knife surgery for trigeminal neuralgia: Detailed analysis of treatment response. *J. Neurosurg.* **2005**, *102*, 442–449. [CrossRef] [PubMed]
11. Régis, J.; Metellus, P.; Hayashi, M.; Roussel, P.; Donnet, A.; Bille-Turc, F. Prospective controlled trial of gamma knife surgery for essential trigeminal neuralgia. *J. Neurosurg.* **2006**, *104*, 913–924. [CrossRef] [PubMed]
12. Zhang, X.; Li, P.; Zhang, S.; Gong, F.; Yang, S.; Wang, W. Effect of radiation dose on the outcomes of gamma knife treatment for trigeminal neuralgia: A multi-factor analysis. *Neurol. India* **2014**, *62*, 400–405. [PubMed]
13. Kim, Y.H.; Kim, D.G.; Kim, J.W.; Han, J.H.; Chung, H.T.; Paek, S.H. Is it effective to raise the irradiation dose from 80 to 85 Gy in gamma knife radiosurgery for trigeminal neuralgia? *Stereotact. Funct. Neurosurg.* **2010**, *88*, 169–176. [CrossRef] [PubMed]

14. Alpert, T.E.; Chung, C.T.; Mitchell, L.T.; Hodge, C.J.; Montgomery, C.T.; Bogart, J.A.; Kim, D.Y.; Bassano, D.A.; Hahn, S.S. Gamma knife surgery for trigeminal neuralgia: improved initial response with two isocenters and increasing dose. *J. Neurosurg.* **2005**, *102*, 185–188. [CrossRef] [PubMed]
15. Longhi, M.; Rizzo, P.; Nicolato, A.; Foroni, R.; Reggio, M.; Gerosa, M. Gamma knife radiosurgery for trigeminal neuralgia: results and potentially predictive parameters—Part I: Idiopathic trigeminal neuralgia. *Neurosurgery* **2007**, *61*, 1254–1260. [CrossRef] [PubMed]
16. Matsuda, S.; Serizawa, T.; Nagano, O.; Ono, J. Comparison of the results of 2 targeting methods in Gamma Knife surgery for trigeminal neuralgia. *J. Neurosurg.* **2008**, *109*, 185–189. [CrossRef] [PubMed]
17. Smith, Z.A.; Gorgulho, A.A.; Bezrukiy, N.; McArthur, D.; Agazaryan, N.; Selch, M.T.; De Salles, A.A. Dedicated linear accelerator radiosurgery for trigeminal neuralgia: A single-center experience in 179 patients with varied dose prescriptions and treatment plans. *Int. J. Radiat. Oncol. Biol. Phys.* **2011**, *81*, 225–231. [CrossRef] [PubMed]
18. Morbidini-Gaffney, S.; Chung, C.T.; Alpert, T.E.; Newman, N.; Hahn, S.S.; Shah, H.; Mitchell, L.; Bassano, D.; Darbar, A.; Bajwa, S.A.; et al. Doses greater than 85 Gy and two isocenters in Gamma Knife surgery for trigeminal neuralgia: Updated results. *J. Neurosurg.* **2006**, *105*, 107–111. [CrossRef]
19. Kotecha, R.; Kotecha, R.; Modugula, S.; Murphy, E.S.; Jones, M.; Kotecha, R.; Reddy, C.A.; Suh, J.H.; Barnett, G.H.; Neyman, G.; et al. Trigeminal Neuralgia Treated with Stereotactic Radiosurgery: The Effect of Dose Escalation on Pain Control and Treatment Outcomes. *Int. J. Radiat. Oncol. Biol. Phys.* **2016**, *96*, 142–148. [CrossRef]
20. Massager, N.; Murata, N.; Tamura, M.; Devriendt, D.; Levivier, M.; Régis, J. Influence of nerve radiation dose in the incidence of trigeminal dysfunction after trigeminal neuralgia radiosurgery. *Neurosurgery* **2007**, *60*, 681–687. [CrossRef]
21. Villavicencio, A.T.; Lim, M.; Burneikiene, S.; Romanelli, P.; Adler, J.R.; McNeely, L.; Chang, S.D.; Fariselli, L.; McIntyre, M.; Bower, R.; et al. Cyberknife radiosurgery for trigeminal neuralgia treatment: A preliminary multicenter experience. *Neurosurgery* **2008**, *62*, 647–655. [CrossRef] [PubMed]
22. Young, B.; Shivazad, A.; Kryscio, R.J.; St Clair, W.; Bush, H.M. Long-term outcome of high-dose γ knife surgery in treatment of trigeminal neuralgia. *J. Neurosurg.* **2013**, *119*, 1166–1175. [CrossRef] [PubMed]
23. Pollock, B.E.; Phuong, L.K.; Gorman, D.A.; Foote, R.L.; Stafford, S.L. Stereotactic radiosurgery for idiopathic trigeminal neuralgia. *J. Neurosurg.* **2002**, *97*, 347–353. [CrossRef] [PubMed]
24. Taich, Z.J.; Goetsch, S.J.; Monaco, E.; Carter, B.S.; Ott, K.; Alksne, J.F.; Chen, C.C. Stereotactic Radiosurgery Treatment of Trigeminal Neuralgia: Clinical Outcomes and Prognostic Factors. *World Neurosurg* **2016**, *90*, 604–612. [CrossRef] [PubMed]
25. Park, S.H.; Hwang, S.K.; Kang, D.H.; Park, J.; Hwang, J.H.; Sung, J.K. The retrogasserian zone versus dorsal root entry zone: comparison of two targeting techniques of gamma knife radiosurgery for trigeminal neuralgia. *Acta Neurochir.* **2010**, *152*, 1165–1170. [CrossRef] [PubMed]
26. Rashid, A.; Pintea, B.; Kinfe, T.M.; Surber, G.; Hamm, K.; Boström, J.P. LINAC stereotactic radiosurgery for trigeminal neuralgia-retrospective two-institutional examination of treatment outcomes. *Radiat. Oncol.* **2018**, *13*, 153. [CrossRef]
27. Xu, Z.; Schlesinger, D.; Moldovan, K.; Przybylowski, C.; Sun, X.; Lee, C.C.; Yen, C.P.; Sheehan, J. Impact of target location on the response of trigeminal neuralgia to stereotactic radiosurgery. *J. Neurosurg.* **2014**, *120*, 716–724. [CrossRef]
28. Sharim, J.; Lo, W.L.; Kim, W.; Chivukula, S.; Tenn, S.; Kaprealian, T.; Pouratian, N. Radiosurgical target distance from the root entry zone in the treatment of trigeminal neuralgia. *Pract. Radiat. Oncol.* **2017**, *7*, 221–227. [CrossRef]
29. Régis, J. High–dose trigeminal neuralgia radiosurgery associated with increased risk of trigeminal nerve dysfunction. *Neurosurgery* **2002**, *50*, 1401–1402.
30. Tuleasca, C.; Régis, J.; Sahgal, A.; De Salles, A.; Hayashi, M.; Ma, L.; Martínez–Álvarez, R.; Paddick, I.; Ryu, S.; Slotman, B.J.; et al. Stereotactic radiosurgery for trigeminal neuralgia: A systematic review International Stereotactic Radiosurgery Society practice guidelines. *J. Neurosurg.* **2019**, *130*, 733–757. [CrossRef]
31. Flickinger, J.C.; Pollock, B.E.; Kondziolka, D.; Phuong, L.K.; Foote, R.L.; Stafford, S.L.; Lunsford, L.D. Does increased nerve length within the treatment volume improve trigeminal neuralgia radiosurgery? A prospective double-blind, randomized study. *Int. J. Radiat. Oncol. Biol. Phys.* **2001**, *51*, 449–454. [CrossRef]

32. Zhao, H.; Shen, Y.; Yao, D.; Xiong, N.; Abdelmaksoud, A.; Wang, H. Outcomes of Two-Isocenter Gamma Knife Radiosurgery for Patients with Typical Trigeminal Neuralgia: Pain Response and Quality of Life. *World Neurosurg.* **2018**, *109*, e531–e538. [CrossRef] [PubMed]
33. Wolf, A.; Tyburczy, A.; Ye, J.C.; Fatterpekar, G.; Silverman, J.S.; Kondziolka, D. The relationship of dose to nerve volume in predicting pain recurrence after stereotactic radiosurgery in trigeminal neuralgia. *J. Neurosurg.* **2018**, *128*, 891–896. [CrossRef] [PubMed]
34. Debono, B.; Lotterie, J.A.; Sol, J.C.; Bousquet, P.; Duthil, P.; Monfraix, S.; Lazorthes, Y.; Sabatier, J.; Latorzeff, I. Dedicated Linear Accelerator Radiosurgery for Classic Trigeminal Neuralgia: A Single–Center Experience with Long-Term Follow-Up. *World Neurosurg.* **2019**, *121*, e775–e785. [CrossRef] [PubMed]
35. Lopez, B.C.; Hamlyn, P.J.; Zakrzewska, J.M. Stereotactic radiosurgery for primary trigeminal neuralgia: state of the evidence and recommendations for future reports. *J. Neurol. Neurosurg. Psychiatry* **2004**, *75*, 1019–1024. [CrossRef] [PubMed]
36. Régis, J.; Carron, R.; Park, M. Is radiosurgery a neuromodulation therapy? A 2009 Fabrikant award lecture. *J. Neurooncol.* **2010**, *98*, 155–162. [CrossRef] [PubMed]
37. Nugent, G.R. Technique and results of 800 percutaneous radiofrequency thermocoagulations for trigeminal neuralgia. *Appl. Neurophysiol.* **1982**, *45*, 504–507. [PubMed]
38. Pollock, B.E. Radiosurgery for trigeminal neuralgia: Is sensory disturbance required for pain relief? *J. Neurosurg.* **2006**, *105*, 103–106. [CrossRef]
39. Kondziolka, D.; Lacomis, D.; Niranjan, A.; Mori, Y.; Maesawa, S.; Fellows, W.; Lunsford, L.D. Histological effects of trigeminal nerve radiosurgery in a primate model: Implications for trigeminal neuralgia radiosurgery. *Neurosurgery* **2000**, *46*, 971–976.
40. Zhao, Z.F.; Yang, L.Z.; Jiang, C.L.; Zheng, Y.R.; Zhang, J.W. Gamma Knife irradiation–induced histopathological changes in the trigeminal nerves of rhesus monkeys. *J. Neurosurg.* **2010**, *113*, 39–44. [CrossRef]

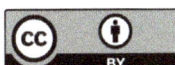

© 2019 by the authors. Licensee MDPI, Basel, Switzerland. This article is an open access article distributed under the terms and conditions of the Creative Commons Attribution (CC BY) license (http://creativecommons.org/licenses/by/4.0/).

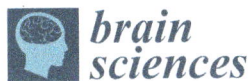

Communication

Adjunct Diagnostic Value of Transcranial Magnetic Stimulation in Mucopolysaccharidosis-Related Cervical Myelopathy: A Pilot Study

Mariagiovanna Cantone [1], Giuseppe Lanza [2,3,*], Alice Le Pira [4], Rita Barone [5], Giovanni Pennisi [2], Rita Bella [6], Manuela Pennisi [7] and Agata Fiumara [4]

1. Department of Neurology, Sant'Elia Hospital, ASP Caltanissetta, Via Luigi Russo 6, 93100 Caltanissetta, Italy
2. Department of Surgery and Medical-Surgical Specialties, University of Catania, Via Santa Sofia 78, 95125 Catania, Italy
3. Department of Neurology IC, Oasi Research Institute—IRCCS, Via Conte Ruggero 73, 94018 Troina, Italy
4. Referral Center for Inherited Metabolic Diseases, Department of Clinical and Experimental Medicine, University of Catania. Via Santa Sofia 78, 95125 Catania, Italy
5. Child Neurology and Psychiatry, Department of Clinical and Experimental Medicine, University of Catania, Via Santa Sofia 78, 95125 Catania, Italy
6. Department of Medical and Surgical Sciences and Advanced Technologies, Section of Neurosciences, University of Catania, Via Santa Sofia 78, 95125 Catania, Italy
7. Department of Biological and Biotechnological Sciences, University of Catania, Via Santa Sofia 78, 95125 Catania, Italy
* Correspondence: glanza@oasi.en.it; Tel.: +39-095-378-2448

Received: 28 June 2019; Accepted: 10 August 2019; Published: 14 August 2019

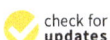

Abstract: Background: Cervical myelopathy (CM) is a common cause of morbidity and disability in patients with mucopolysaccharidosis (MPS) and, therefore, early detection is crucial for the best surgical intervention and follow-up. Transcranial magnetic stimulation (TMS) non-invasively evaluates the conduction through the cortico-spinal tract, also allowing preclinical diagnosis and monitoring. Methods: Motor evoked potentials (MEPs) to TMS were recorded in a group of eight patients with MPS-related CM. Responses were obtained during mild tonic muscular activation by means of a circular coil held on the "hot spot" of the first dorsal interosseous and tibialis anterior muscles, bilaterally. The motor latency by cervical or lumbar magnetic stimulation was subtracted from the MEP cortical latency to obtain the central motor conduction time. The MEP amplitude from peak to peak to cortical stimulation and the interside difference of each measure were also calculated. Results: TMS revealed abnormal findings from both upper and lower limbs compatible with axonal damage and demyelination in six of them. Notably, a subclinical cervical spinal disease was detected before the occurrence of an overt CM in two patients, whereas TMS signs compatible with a CM of variable degree persisted despite surgery in all treated subjects. Conclusions: TMS can be viewed as an adjunct diagnostic test pending further rigorous investigations.

Keywords: motor evoked potentials lysosomal disorders; cortical-spinal tract; spinal cord compression; cervical myelopathy; clinical neurophysiology

1. Introduction

1.1. Mucopolysaccharidosis: A Brief Overview

Mucopolysaccharidosis (MPS) encompasses a group of inherited rare lysosomal diseases due to defective catabolism and storage of glycosaminoglycans (GAG) in the skeleton and soft tissues. MPS shows a wide and heterogeneous spectrum of clinical manifestations and severity, ranging from severe to very mild phenotypes that may be recognized only in adulthood. Diagnosis is based on the demonstration of elevated urinary excretion of mucopolysaccharides, enzyme deficiency, and genetic testing [1]. Enzyme replacement therapy (ERT) is available for MPS I, II, IVA, VI, and VII.

MPS I (Hurler or Scheie syndrome) and type II (Hunter syndrome) are the most common MPS types. The typical presentation is a pre-school age patient with developmental delay, short stature, recurrent ear and respiratory infections, and hepato-splenomegaly. Over time, the child develops hearing loss, cardiac valve disease, airway obstruction, skeletal contractures, distinctive facial appearance (macrocephaly, thick eyebrows, gingival hypertrophy, macroglossia, thickening of the lips and nasal alae), psycho-motor regression, and intellectual disability [1,2]. The characteristic radiographic findings, collectively termed dysostosis multiplex, include J-shaped sella turcica, oar-shaped ribs, pointing of the proximal metacarpals and metatarsals, and poorly developed acetabulum [3]. Untreated, the life expectancy is the second or third decade. Milder forms of MPS I and II have less prominent somatic findings and no CNS disease or intellectual disability [4].

MPS III is characterized by the predominance of neuropsychiatric rather than somatic problems, with developmental delay and intellectual disability manifesting early on [2]. In severe cases, development plateaus between 36 and 40 months, and these patients never learn to speak more than a few single words [5,6]. As the disease progresses, significant cognitive-behavioral (aggression, hyperactivity, decreased attention span, anxiety, and destructive behaviors) and sleep disturbances (difficulty falling asleep and frequent nighttime wakening) occur [5]. The progressive GAG deposition in the brain leads to seizures, spasticity, and feeding difficulties, gradually causing loss of language and ambulation till a vegetative state [4].

MPS IV (Morquio syndrome) includes type A and B, which are difficult to distinguish clinically, although the former is far more common. The age of onset is generally in the first few years of life [1]. Clinical manifestations are: short stature, pectus carinatum, forearm deformity, genu valgum, scoliosis, hip dysplasia, odontoid hypoplasia with atlanto-axial instability, and dental abnormalities. Non-skeletal features include corneal clouding, hearing loss, obstructive or restrictive lung disease, and cardiac dysfunction, whereas the intellect is normal [4]. A considerable spectrum of severity exists, and mildly affected individuals may have normal height and few clinical complications [7].

MPS VI (Maroteaux-Lamy syndrome) is characterized by storage of dermatan sulphate, but heparan sulphate metabolism is not impaired and, therefore, the intellect is generally normal [1]. This type shares many of the features of MPS I and II, including short stature, coarse facies, corneal clouding, airway obstruction, cardiac valve abnormalities, visceromegaly, inguinal and umbilical hernias, dysostosis multiplex, joint contractures, carpal tunnel syndrome, and hip dysplasia. The age of onset and disease progression are variable [4].

MPS VII is an ultra-rare disease. Notably, 40–45% of patients present with non-immune fetal hydrops [8,9], which is considered a relatively suggestive finding for MPS VII. In patients who survive beyond the neonatal period, common clinical features include intellectual disability, coarse facies, dysostosis multiplex, joint contractures, hepato-splenomegaly, scoliosis, corneal clouding, obstructive airway disease, cardiac valve disease, and cardiomyopathy [8].

1.2. Cervical Myelopathy in MPS

Cervical myelopathy (CM) is most frequently observed in MPS I, II, IV, and VI. It is the main cause of neurological morbidity and disability in these patients [10], with a significantly negative impact on their course of disease and quality of life [11]. CM is due to vertebral canal narrowing, which often results from the thickening of the dura mater and ligaments after GAG accumulation and fibrosis, epidural lipomatosis, and vertebral soma degeneration. Atlanto-axial subluxation due to odontoid hypoplasia may contribute to spinal cord compression and related clinical manifestations.

Although the effectiveness of ERT has been proven on different systemic complications of MPS, thus improving the lifespan of these patients, it does not have any effect on CM [12]. Given that an early detection of CM is associated with the best surgical outcome and post-operative course, both an accurate diagnosis and strict monitoring are recommended [13].

Magnetic resonance imaging (MRI) and computed tomography are the methods of choice to display spinal cord compression and vertebral abnormalities, respectively, although they do not provide any information on the functional status. In this context, motor evoked potentials (MEPs) to Transcranial Magnetic Stimulation (TMS) are diffusely used in clinical practice for the in vivo and real time non-invasive estimation of the excitation state and conduction velocity of the cortico-spinal tract [14], also allowing a preclinical diagnosis and monitoring [15–22]. In particular, MEP latency and central motor conduction time (CMCT) are viewed as reliable measures of the cortical-spinal myelination, whereas the MEP amplitude is known to reflect the status of excitation of the neuronal axons from the motor cortical areas to the spinal motoneurons till the muscles [14].

While several and robust TMS evidences are available in patients with different neurological disorders affecting the central motor system, to date few neurophysiological studies have been carried out in MPS-related CM [23–27]. Here, we applied TMS in patients with MPS to detect any electrophysiological sign, even at a subclinical level, of CM.

2. Materials and Methods

2.1. Subjects and Assessment

Eight patients (two males; median age 14.5 years, range 13.0–41.0) with a clinical, biochemical, and genetic diagnosis of MPS [28] were consecutively recruited from the "Referral Center for Inherited Metabolic Diseases, Department of Clinical and Experimental Medicine" of the University of Catania, Italy. Among these subjects, six (patient 1–6) had MPS IVA, whereas the remaining two (patient 7 and 8) had MPS VI.

As shown in Table 1, six subjects (1–4, 7, and 8) had previously received surgical decompression due to clinical and MRI evidence of CM, although four of them (1, 3, 7, and 8) still complained of neurological deficits. Regardless of previous surgery, at the time of the study, four patients with MPS IVA (2, 4, 5, and 6) did not have radiological evidences of CM. Finally, the two subjects with MPS VI had been treated with ERT for three years. The cervical cord compression and the CM at MRI were diagnosed by a trained neuroradiologist expert in vertebral and spinal cord diseases.

Table 1. Clinical and demographic characteristics of MPS patients at the time of the study.

Patient	1	2	3	4	5	6	7	8
MPS type	IVA	IVA	IVA	IVA	IVA	IVA	VI	VI
Sex/age (years)	F/14	M/15	F/16	M/13	F/20	F/40	F/13	F/14
ERT (age, years)	-	-	-	-	-	-	+ (9)	+ (10)
Height (cm)	98	100	102	110	150	113	120	110
Spinal cord surgery (age, years)	+ (5)	+ (4)	+ (8)	+ (10)	-	-	+ (10)	+ (11)
Diffuse brisk tendon reflex	+	-	+	+	-	-	+	+
Limbs paresis/weakness	+	-	+	-	-	-	+	+
Walking assistance	+	-	+	-	-	-	-	+
MRI cervical cord compression	+	+	+	+	-	-	+	+
MRI cervical myelopathy	+	-	+	-	-	-	-	+

MPS = mucopolysaccharidosis; F = female; M = male; ERT = enzyme replacement therapy; MRI = magnetic resonance imaging; + = present; - = absent.

This research was performed according to the Declaration of Helsinki and all participants (or parents) gave their informed consent for inclusion before they participated in the study. This investigation was part of a larger multi-center study on clinical and molecular characterization of patients with MPS. The Ethics Committee of the "Azienda Ospedaliero-Universitaria Policlinico—Vittorio Emanuele" of Catania, Italy (PRIN 2012 code 20122EK9SZ_005) approved the study.

2.2. Transcranial Magnetic Stimulation

MEPs to TMS is included within the conventional diagnostic work-up of patients with suspected or overt CM, as well as in the peri- and post-operative course [14].

For diagnostic TMS, a high-power MagStim 220 mono-pulse stimulator (The Magstim Co., Ltd., Whitland, Dyfed, UK) connected to a 90 mm circular coil with an inner diameter of 5 cm, was employed to generate the motor responses. In a conventional exam, the patient is seated or lying on an armchair while recordings from distal limb muscles are performed. Standard EMG silver/silver chloride cup surface electrodes (9 mm diameter), jelly filled and applied over the first dorsal interosseous (FDI) and tibialis anterior (TA) muscles in a conventional belly tendon montage, were used for MEPs recordings from the contralateral side of stimulation [14].

The handle of the coil was pointing backward, whereas the coil center was positioned tangentially over Cz (international EEG 10–20 system) for MEP recordings from the FDI muscle and over Fz for MEP recordings from the TA muscle. A MEP to TMS in the relaxed muscle was first recorded. After that, MEPs with higher amplitude and shorter latency compared to the first response were obtained while patients produced a transient tonic muscular activity just enough to overcome gravity (approximately 10–20% of the maximal muscular activity). According to international guidelines, the shortest MEP latency was used for CMCT estimation. Similarly, only the MEP with the largest peak-to-peak size was considered for the analysis, given that a routine TMS exam evaluates the transcranially-induced motor response with the biggest amplitude. To determine the peripheral motor conduction time (PMCT), a motor nerve root stimulation was performed in all participants. The coil center was applied on the 7th cervical and 4th lumbar spinous process for upper and lower limbs, respectively. The time of conduction from the neurons within the motor cortex to those within the anterior horn of the spinal cord defines the CMCT, thus reflecting the central motor conductivity from the upper to the lower motoneuron. The PMCT by cervical or lumbar magnetic stimulation was subtracted from the MEP cortical latency to obtain the CMCT [14].

Given that the stimulation threshold for a 2.0 T magnetic stimulator (as that used in this study) is about 50–65% of the maximal output [29–31], motor responses were all obtained at 80% of the maximum stimulator output. The amplification and filtering (bandwidth 3–3000 Hz) of the motor responses were carried out by using a 2-channel Medelec Synergy system (Oxford Instruments Medical, Inc., Surrey, UK). As reference MEP values, we referred to those used in our TMS Lab, which were obtained from a large cohort of clinically and neuroradiologically intact subjects divided by age, height, and sex [32].

3. Results

Table 2 summarizes the patients' neurophysiological features. Overall, TMS was well tolerated and none complained of significant side-effects or discomfort during or after the examination. Figure 1 shows examples of both normal and pathological MEP recordings.

Among those who had underwent surgery for CM (patient 1–4, 7, and 8), MEPs were bilaterally absent from FDI and TA muscles in both patients with MPS VI (7 and 8), who already had a neurological impairment before treatment. In the treated patients with MPS IVA (1–4), MEPs were bilaterally absent from TA muscle in patient 3 as well as from the left TA muscle of patient 1. In the same patients (1–4), MEPs also showed reduced amplitude and polyphasic shape. Overall, CMCT was increased in three of the treated subjects from upper limbs (1, 2, and 4), whereas responses to cervical root stimulation could not be evoked in the other three (3, 7, and 8).

Regarding the four subjects without overt neurological symptoms (2, 4, 5, and 6), MEPs were abnormal in terms of reduced amplitude, increased latency, or polyphasic shape in at least one of the examined muscles in two of them (patient 2 and 4), whereas they were entirely normal in the other two (patient 5 and 6).

Table 2. Motor evoked potentials of MPS patients.

	First Dorsal Interosseous Muscle											Tibialis Anterior Muscle								
	MEPs Amp (mV)			Poly-Phasic Shape		MEPs Latency (ms)			CMCT (ms)			MEPs Amp (mV)			MEPs Latency (ms)			CMCT (ms)		
N	R	L	ID	R	L	R	L	ID	R	L	ID	R	L	ID	R	L	ID	R	L	ID
	>2.8	>2.8	<4.0	-	-	<22.5	<22.5	<1.5	<7.6	<7.6	<1.5	>1.9	>1.9	<4.0	<31.2	<31.2	<4.1	<17.2	<17.2	<3.0
1	0.2	0.1	0.1	-	+	19.2	20.0	0.8	nr	10.1	/	0.3	nr	/	29.3	nr	/	21.2	nr	/
2	2.6	2.2	0.4	+	-	16.5	17.1	0.6	8.1	8.1	0.0	3.2	1.7	1.5	19.6	21.5	1.9	12.3	14.0	1.7
3	0.3	0.2	0.1	+	+	19.4	20.6	1.2	nr	nr	/	nr	nr	/	nr	nr	/	nr	nr	/
4	0.8	0.6	0.2	+	+	17.3	17.2	0.1	9.6	9.4	0.2	2.9	2.5	0.4	18.5	19.8	1.3	12.5	12.6	0.1
5	8.0	7.0	1.0	-	-	17.4	16.2	1.2	5.4	6.0	0.6	7.0	6.0	1.0	20.0	19.5	0.5	11.6	11.6	0.0
6	3.8	3.5	0.3	-	-	18.3	18.5	0.2	6.1	6.4	0.3	3.0	4.0	1.0	24.9	25.2	0.3	14.7	14.3	0.4
7	nr	nr	/	/	/	nr	nr	/	nr	nr	/	nr	nr	/	nr	nr	/	nr	nr	/
8	nr	nr	/	/	/	nr	nr	/	nr	nr	/	nr	nr	/	nr	nr	/	nr	nr	/

MPS = mucopolysaccharidosis; N = patient number; MEPs = motor evoked potentials; R = right; L = left; ID = interside difference; - = absent; + = present; amp = amplitude; CMCT = central motor conduction time; nr = value not recordable due to the absence of the transcranially-induced motor response (MEP latency column) or the absence of the response by cervical or lumbar nerve root stimulation (CMCT column); numbers in italics = reference values [32]; numbers in bold = pathological values.

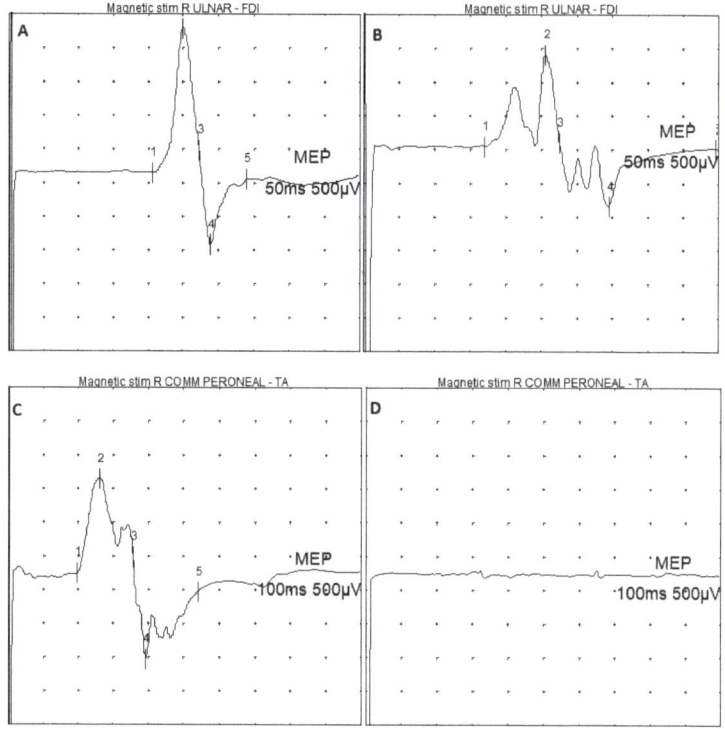

Figure 1. Examples of MEPs recordings in MPS patients. (**A**) normal MEP from the upper limb; (**B**) MEP with reduced amplitude and polyphasic shape from the upper limb; (**C**) normal MEP from the lower limb; (**D**) absence of transcranially-induced motor response from the lower limb. MPS = mucopolysaccharidosis; Magnetic stim = transcranial magnetic stimulation; R ULNAR = right ulnar nerve; R COMM PERONEAL = right common peroneal nerve; FDI = first dorsal interosseous muscle; TA = tibialis anterior muscle; MEP = motor evoked potential; 50 ms = temporal resolution of the screen (sweep) for upper limb recordings; 100 ms = temporal resolution of the screen (sweep) for lower limb recordings; 500 µV = amplification factor of the screen.

CMCT could not be bilaterally assessed at four limbs in three patients (3, 7, and 8) due to the absence of the evoked response by cervical or lumbar nerve root magnetic stimulation. Finally, no significant right-to-left difference was found for any of the TMS variables considered.

4. Discussion

In the present study, we found abnormal TMS findings from upper and/or lower limbs in six out of eight MPS patients, consistent with both diffuse axonal damage and demyelination. This suggests that a cervical spinal disease was clinically present before the occurrence of an overt CM and persisted, with a different clinical and neurophysiological level of severity, despite surgery. In this context, it should be acknowledged that patients with MPS may suffer from a wide spectrum of neurological symptoms that involves both CNS and the peripheral nerves and the musculo-skeletal system. In particular, they usually need neurosurgical intervention for CM or vertebro-spinal anomalies, although a spinal cord compression may occur and progress even in the absence of overt neurological symptoms [33].

Notably, MEPs response were bilaterally absent at four limbs from the two patients with MPS VI. This finding is compatible with a severe CM-related involvement of the cortico-spinal tract and suggests that this MPS type is particularly associated with an early-onset CM and related complications.

Accordingly, recent recommendations from the "MPS VI Clinical Surveillance Program" conclude that patients with MPS VI, even from an early age, are all at high risk to develop CM and that, from the time of the diagnosis, monitoring with MRI should be performed [34]. Moreover, management of peri-operative course of MPS VI patients is often challenging and, therefore, the electrophysiological studies play a significant role in providing both surgical indication and proper timing, as well as in the monitoring of post-operative course. MEPs analysis also revealed a functional impairment even in two patients without a clear evidence of CM, thus allowing a preclinical diagnosis [23]. Therefore, TMS can be viewed as an extension of clinical examination and the functional counterpart of the neuroimaging techniques in assessing spinal cord disease, including the very early stages.

To date, the role of electrophysiological studies in detecting compressive myelopathy in patients with MPS has been investigated by few previous reports [23–25], and one study only has used TMS for the evaluation of the post-operative follow-up in a single patient with MPS VI [23]. In this frame, the intraoperative neurophysiological monitoring by using MEPs and somatosensory evoked potentials seems to be of pivotal interest as it provides relevant functional information during surgical procedures [27]. Since cervical cord compression in MPS is progressive and may produce rapid loss of sensory-motor functions in these patients (especially in those with type VI), surgery is indicated as soon as myelopathy is detected, even subclinically, as severely myelopathic subjects show little or no recovery after the operation [24,35], also at the TMS level, as confirmed by the present investigation.

It is worthwhile to mention that histological examination in a mice model of MPS type I showed a storage of GAG in the cortex and cerebellum, along with the evidence of a progressive inflammatory response that can contribute to the neurological deficit [36]. Based on its intrinsic properties, TMS might be considered as an additional tool able to disclose subclinical CNS involvement related to a neuroinflammatory status in MPS, a finding which has also been demonstrated in other autoimmune and metabolic disorders [37–39]. In this view, innovative neuromodulatory protocols based on non-invasive brain stimulation techniques might be applied to transiently modulate cortical excitability, synaptic plasticity, and functional connectivity [40–44].

The main limitation of this study is the small sample size, although MPS is a rare disorder. Nevertheless, these findings have to be interpreted with caution, since the small and heterogeneous data set does not allow to draw definite conclusions. Another caveat is that only patients with severe MPS VI phenotype were included, thus we cannot compare these findings with those from patients with mild phenotype. Finally, long term MEP data, before and after surgical intervention, are needed to confirm the role of TMS for prognostication purposes. Therefore, the results provided here should be considered descriptive and to be used as an adjunct test pending further rigorous investigations. Future studies and longitudinal exams are needed for early diagnosis, accurate prognosis, and adequate monitoring.

Author Contributions: Conceptualization, M.C. and R.B. (Rita Barone); methodology, G.L.; validation, A.L.P., A.F., and M.P.; formal analysis, G.P.; investigation, R.B. (Rita Barone); data curation, R.B. (Rita Bella); writing—original draft preparation, M.C. and G.L.; writing—review and editing, A.L.P. and M.P.; visualization, A.F.; supervision, R.B. (Rita Bella); project administration, G.P.; All authors approved the submitted version and agreed to be personally accountable for the author's own contributions and for ensuring that questions related to the accuracy or integrity of any part of the work.

Funding: This study was supported by the Italian MIUR (Ministero dell'Istruzione, dell' Università e della Ricerca), for the "PRIN 2012 National Research Program" project (Prot. 20122EK9SZ_002) entitled "Comprehensive approach to mucopolysaccharidoses: application of highly specific methods for neonatal diagnosis and assessment of therapeutic efficacy in patients and in experimental animals".

Conflicts of Interest: The authors declare no conflict of interest.

References

1. Stapleton, M.; Arunkumar, N.; Kubaski, F.; Mason, R.W.; Tadao, O.; Tomatsu, S. Clinical presentation and diagnosis of mucopolysaccharidoses. *Mol. Genet. Metab.* **2018**, *125*, 4–17. [CrossRef] [PubMed]

2. Barone, R.; Pellico, A.; Pittalà, A.; Gasperini, S. Neurobehavioral phenotypes of neuronopathic mucopolysaccharidoses. *Ital. J. Pediatr.* **2018**, *44*, 121. [CrossRef] [PubMed]
3. Palmucci, S.; Attinà, G.; Lanza, M.L.; Belfiore, G.; Cappello, G.; Foti, P.V.; Milone, P.; Di Bella, D.; Barone, R.; Fiumara, A.; et al. Imaging findings of mucopolysaccharidoses: A pictorial review. *Insights Imaging* **2013**, *4*, 443–459. [CrossRef] [PubMed]
4. Sun, A. Lysosomal storage disease overview. *Ann. Transl. Med.* **2018**, *6*, 476. [CrossRef] [PubMed]
5. Valstar, M.J.; Neijs, S.; Bruggenwirth, H.T.; Olmer, R.; Ruijter, G.J.; Wevers, R.A.; van Diggelen, O.P.; Poorthuis, B.J.; Halley, D.J.; Wijburg, F.A. Mucopolysaccharidosis type IIIA: Clinical spectrum and genotype-phenotype correlations. *Ann. Neurol.* **2010**, *68*, 876–887. [CrossRef] [PubMed]
6. Shapiro, E.G.; Nestrasil, I.; Delaney, K.A.; Rudser, K.; Kovac, V.; Nair, N.; Richard, C.W., 3rd; Haslett, P.; Whitley, C.B. A Prospective Natural History Study of Mucopolysaccharidosis Type IIIA. *J. Pediatr.* **2016**, *170*, e1–e4. [CrossRef] [PubMed]
7. Hendriksz, C.J.; Harmatz, P.; Beck, M.; Jones, S.; Wood, T.; Lachman, R.; Gravance, C.G.; Orii, T.; Tomatsu, S. Review of clinical presentation and diagnosis of mucopolysaccharidosis IVA. *Mol. Genet. Metab.* **2013**, *110*, 54–64. [CrossRef] [PubMed]
8. Montaño, A.M.; Lock-Hock, N.; Steiner, R.D.; Graham, B.H.; Szlago, M.; Greenstein, R.; Pineda, M.; Gonzalez-Meneses, A.; Çoker, M.; Bartholomew, D.; et al. Clinical course of sly syndrome (mucopolysaccharidosis type VII). *J. Med. Genet.* **2016**, *53*, 403–418. [CrossRef] [PubMed]
9. Zielonka, M.; Garbade, S.F.; Kölker, S.; Hoffmann, G.F.; Ries, M. Quantitative clinical characteristics of 53 patients with MPS VII: A cross-sectional analysis. *Genet. Med.* **2018**, *20*, 474. [CrossRef]
10. Galimberti, C.; Madeo, A.; Di Rocco, M.; Fiumara, A. Mucopolysaccharidoses: Early diagnostic signs in infants and children. *Ital. J. Pediatr.* **2018**, *44*, 133. [CrossRef]
11. Giussani, C.; Guida, L.; Canonico, F.; Sganzerla, E.P. Cerebral and occipito-atlanto-axial involvement in mucopolysaccharidosis patients: Clinical, radiological, and neurosurgical features. *Ital. J. Pediatr.* **2018**, *44*, 119. [CrossRef] [PubMed]
12. Illsinger, S.; Lücke, T.; Hartmann, H.; Mengel, E.; Müller-Forell, W.; Donnerstag, F.; Das, A.M. Scheie syndrome: Enzyme replacement therapy does not prevent progression of cervical myelopathy due to spinal cord compression. *J. Inherit. Metab. Dis.* **2009**, *32*, 321–325. [CrossRef] [PubMed]
13. Solanki, G.A.; Martin, K.W.; Theroux, M.C.; Lampe, C.; White, K.K.; Shediac, R.; Lampe, C.G.; Beck, M.; Mackenzie, W.G.; Hendriksz, C.J.; et al. Spinal involvement in mucopolysaccharidosis IVA (Morquio-Brailsford or Morquio A syndrome): Presentation, diagnosis and management. *J. Inherit. Metab. Dis.* **2013**, *36*, 339–355. [CrossRef] [PubMed]
14. Rossini, P.M.; Burke, D.; Chen, R.; Cohen, L.G.; Daskalakis, Z.; Di Iorio, R.; Di Lazzaro, V.; Ferreri, F.; Fitzgerald, P.B.; George, M.S.; et al. Non-invasive electrical and magnetic stimulation of the brain, spinal cord, roots and peripheral nerves: Basic principles and procedures for routine clinical and research application. An updated report from an I.F.C.N. Committee. *Clin. Neurophysiol.* **2015**, *126*, 1071–1107. [CrossRef] [PubMed]
15. Travlos, A.; Pant, B.; Eisen, A. Transcranial magnetic stimulation for detection of preclinical cervical spondylotic myelopathy. *Arch. Phys. Med. Rehabil.* **1992**, *73*, 442–446. [PubMed]
16. Bella, R.; Ferri, R.; Cantone, M.; Pennisi, M.; Lanza, G.; Malaguarnera, G.; Spampinato, C.; Giordano, D.; Raggi, A.; Pennisi, G. Motor cortex excitability in vascular depression. *Int. J. Psychophysiol.* **2011**, *82*, 248–253. [CrossRef] [PubMed]
17. Lanza, G.; Bella, R.; Giuffrida, S.; Cantone, M.; Pennisi, G.; Spampinato, C.; Giordano, D.; Malaguarnera, G.; Raggi, A.; Pennisi, M. Preserved transcallosal inhibition to transcranial magnetic stimulation in nondemented elderly patients with leukoaraiosis. *Biomed. Res. Int.* **2013**, *2013*, 351680. [CrossRef] [PubMed]
18. Bella, R.; Ferri, R.; Lanza, G.; Cantone, M.; Pennisi, M.; Puglisi, V.; Vinciguerra, L.; Spampinato, C.; Mazza, T.; Malaguarnera, G.; et al. TMS follow-up study in patients with vascular cognitive impairment-no dementia. *Neurosci. Lett.* **2013**, *534*, 155–159. [CrossRef] [PubMed]
19. Pennisi, G.; Bella, R.; Lanza, G. Motor cortex plasticity in subcortical ischemic vascular dementia: What can TMS say? *Clin. Neurophysiol.* **2015**, *126*, 851–852. [CrossRef]
20. Bella, R.; Cantone, M.; Lanza, G.; Ferri, R.; Vinciguerra, L.; Puglisi, V.; Pennisi, M.; Ricceri, R.; Di Lazzaro, V.; Pennisi, G. Cholinergic circuitry functioning in patients with vascular cognitive impairment–no dementia. *Brain Stimul.* **2016**, *9*, 225–233. [CrossRef]

21. Lanza, G.; Bramanti, P.; Cantone, M.; Pennisi, M.; Pennisi, G.; Bella, R. Vascular Cognitive Impairment through the Looking Glass of Transcranial Magnetic Stimulation. *Behav. Neurol.* **2017**, *2017*, 1421326. [CrossRef] [PubMed]
22. Cantone, M.; Bramanti, A.; Lanza, G.; Pennisi, M.; Bramanti, P.; Pennisi, G.; Bella, R. Cortical Plasticity in Depression. *ASN Neuro* **2017**, *9*, 1759091417711512. [CrossRef] [PubMed]
23. Boor, R.; Fricke, G.; Brühl, K.; Spranger, J. Abnormal subcortical somatosensory evoked potentials indicate high cervical myelopathy in achondroplasia. *Eur. J. Pediatr.* **1999**, *158*, 662–667. [CrossRef] [PubMed]
24. Boor, R.; Miebach, E.; Brühl, K.; Beck, M. Abnormal somatosensory evoked potentials indicate compressive cervical myelopathy in mucopolysaccharidoses. *Neuropediatrics* **2000**, *31*, 122–127. [CrossRef] [PubMed]
25. Li, L.; Müller-Forell, W.; Oberman, B.; Boor, R. Subcortical somatosensory evoked potentials after median nerve and posterior tibial nerve stimulation in high cervical cord compression of achondroplasia. *Brain Dev.* **2008**, *30*, 499–503. [CrossRef] [PubMed]
26. Mut, M.; Cila, A.; Varli, K.; Akalan, N. Multilevel myelopathy in Maroteaux-Lamy syndrome and review of the literature. *Clin. Neurol. Neurosurg.* **2005**, *107*, 230–235. [CrossRef]
27. Kandil, A.I.; Pettit, C.S.; Berry, L.N.; Busso, V.O.; Careskey, M.; Chesnut, E.; Buck, D.W.; Leslie, N.D.; Tamai, J.; McAuliffe, J.J.; et al. Tertiary Pediatric Academic Institution's Experience With Intraoperative Neuromonitoring for Nonspinal Surgery in Children With Mucopolysaccharidosis, Based on a Novel Evidence-Based Care Algorithm. *Anesth. Analg.* **2019**. [CrossRef]
28. Wraith, J.E. Mucopolysaccharidoses and mucolipidoses. *Handb. Clin. Neurol.* **2013**, *113*, 1723–1729. [CrossRef]
29. Amassian, V.E.; Cracco, R.Q.; Maccabee, P.J. Focal stimulation of human cerebral cortex with the magnetic coil: A comparison with electrical stimulation. *Electroencephalogr. Clin. Neurophysiol.* **1989**, *74*, 401–416. [CrossRef]
30. Alexeeva, N.; Broton, J.G.; Calancie, B. Latency of changes in spinal motoneuron excitability evoked by transcranial magnetic brain stimulation in spinal cord injured individuals. *Electroencephalogr. Clin. Neurophysiol.* **1998**, *109*, 297–303. [CrossRef]
31. Garry, M.I.; Kamen, G.; Nordstrom, M.A. Hemispheric differences in the relationship between corticomotor excitability changes following a fine-motor task and motor learning. *J. Neurophysiol.* **2004**, *91*, 1570–1578. [CrossRef]
32. Cantone, M.; Lanza, G.; Vinciguerra, L.; Puglisi, V.; Ricceri, R.; Fisicaro, F.; Vagli, C.; Bella, R.; Ferri, R.; Pennisi, G.; et al. Age, Height, and Sex on Motor Evoked Potentials: Translational Data From a Large Italian Cohort in a Clinical Environment. *Front. Hum. Neurosci.* **2019**, *13*, 185. [CrossRef]
33. Charrow, J.; Alden, T.D.; Breathnach, C.A.; Frawley, G.P.; Hendriksz, C.J.; Link, B.; Mackenzie, W.G.; Manara, R.; Offiah, A.C.; Solano, M.L.; et al. Diagnostic evaluation, monitoring, and perioperative management of spinal cord compression in patients with Morquio syndrome. *Mol. Genet. Metab.* **2015**, *114*, 11–18. [CrossRef]
34. Solanki, G.A.; Sun, P.P.; Martin, K.W.; Hendriksz, C.J.; Lampe, C.; Guffon, N.; Hung, A.; Sisic, Z.; Shediac, R.; Harmatz, P.R. CSP Study Group.Cervical cord compression in mucopolysaccharidosis VI (MPS VI): Findings from the MPS VI Clinical Surveillance Program (CSP). *Mol. Genet. Metab.* **2016**, *118*, 310–318. [CrossRef]
35. Ransford, A.O.; Crockard, H.A.; Stevens, J.M.; Modaghegh, S. Occipito-atlanto-axial fusion in Morquio-Brailsford syndrome. A ten-year experience. *J. Bone Joint Surg. Br.* **1996**, *78*, 307–313. [CrossRef]
36. Baldo, G.; Mayer, F.Q.; Martinelli, B.; Dilda, A.; Meyer, F.; Ponder, K.P.; Giugliani, R.; Matte, U. Evidence of a progressive motor dysfunction in Mucopolysaccharidosis type I mice. *Behav. Brain Res.* **2012**, *233*, 169–175. [CrossRef]
37. Pennisi, G.; Lanza, G.; Giuffrida, S.; Vinciguerra, L.; Puglisi, V.; Cantone, M.; Pennisi, M.; D'Agate, C.C.; Naso, P.; Aprile, G.; et al. Excitability of the motor cortex in de novo patients with celiac disease. *PLoS ONE* **2014**, *9*, e102790. [CrossRef]
38. Bella, R.; Lanza, G.; Cantone, M.; Giuffrida, S.; Puglisi, V.; Vinciguerra, L.; Pennisi, M.; Ricceri, R.; D'Agate, C.C.; Malaguarnera, G.; et al. Effect of a Gluten-Free Diet on Cortical Excitability in Adults with Celiac Disease. *PLoS ONE* **2015**, *10*, e0129218. [CrossRef]
39. Pennisi, M.; Lanza, G.; Cantone, M.; Ricceri, R.; Ferri, R.; D'Agate, C.C.; Pennisi, G.; Di Lazzaro, V.; Bella, R. Cortical involvement in celiac disease before and after long-term gluten-free diet: A Transcranial Magnetic Stimulation study. *PLoS ONE* **2017**, *12*, e0177560. [CrossRef]

40. Sasso, V.; Bisicchia, E.; Latini, L.; Ghiglieri, V.; Cacace, F.; Carola, V.; Molinari, M.; Viscomi, M.T. Repetitive transcranial magnetic stimulation reduces remote apoptotic cell death and inflammation after focal brain injury. *J. Neuroinflamm.* **2016**, *13*, 150. [CrossRef]
41. Bordet, R.; Ihl, R.; Korczyn, A.D.; Lanza, G.; Jansa, J.; Hoerr, R.; Guekht, A. Towards the concept of disease-modifier in post-stroke or vascular cognitive impairment: A consensus report. *BMC Med.* **2017**, *15*, 107. [CrossRef]
42. Lanza, G.; Cantone, M.; Aricò, D.; Lanuzza, B.; Cosentino, F.I.I.; Paci, D.; Papotto, M.; Pennisi, M.; Bella, R.; Pennisi, G.; et al. Clinical and electrophysiological impact of repetitive low-frequency transcranial magnetic stimulation on the sensory-motor network in patients with restless legs syndrome. *Ther. Adv. Neurol. Disord.* **2018**, *11*, 1756286418759973. [CrossRef]
43. Lanza, G.; Lanuzza, B.; Aricò, D.; Cantone, M.; Cosentino, F.I.I.; Bella, R.; Pennisi, G.; Ferri, R.; Pennisi, M. Impaired short-term plasticity in restless legs syndrome: A pilot rTMS study. *Sleep Med.* **2018**, *46*, 1–4. [CrossRef]
44. Medina-Fernández, F.J.; Escribano, B.M.; Padilla-Del-Campo, C.; Drucker-Colín, R.; Pascual-Leone, A.; Túnez, I. Transcranial magnetic stimulation as an antioxidant. *Free Radic. Res.* **2018**, *52*, 381–389. [CrossRef]

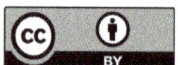 © 2019 by the authors. Licensee MDPI, Basel, Switzerland. This article is an open access article distributed under the terms and conditions of the Creative Commons Attribution (CC BY) license (http://creativecommons.org/licenses/by/4.0/).

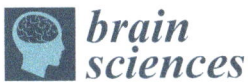

Article

Cellular Changes in Injured Rat Spinal Cord Following Electrical Brainstem Stimulation

Walter J. Jermakowicz [1,*], Stephanie S. Sloley [2], Lia Dan [2], Alberto Vitores [2], Melissa M. Carballosa-Gautam [2] and Ian D. Hentall [2]

[1] Department of Neurological Surgery, University of Miami, 1095 NW 14th Terr., Miami, FL 33136, USA
[2] Miami Project to Cure Paralysis, University of Miami, 1095 NW 14th Terr., Miami, FL 33136, USA; ssloley@gmail.com (S.S.S.); blurryblue@gmail.com (L.D.); alb9402@hotmail.com (A.V.); mcarballosa@gmail.com (M.M.C.-G.); IHentall@med.miami.edu (I.D.H.)
* Correspondence: walter.jermakowicz@jhsmiami.org; Tel.: +1-615-818-3070

Received: 6 May 2019; Accepted: 27 May 2019; Published: 28 May 2019

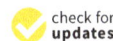

Abstract: Spinal cord injury (SCI) is a major cause of disability and pain, but little progress has been made in its clinical management. Low-frequency electrical stimulation (LFS) of various anti-nociceptive targets improves outcomes after SCI, including motor recovery and mechanical allodynia. However, the mechanisms of these beneficial effects are incompletely delineated and probably multiple. Our aim was to explore near-term effects of LFS in the hindbrain's nucleus raphe magnus (NRM) on cellular proliferation in a rat SCI model. Starting 24 h after incomplete contusional SCI at C5, intermittent LFS at 8 Hz was delivered wirelessly to NRM. Controls were given inactive stimulators. At 48 h, 5-bromodeoxyuridine (BrdU) was administered and, at 72 h, spinal cords were extracted and immunostained for various immune and neuroglial progenitor markers and BrdU at the level of the lesion and proximally and distally. LFS altered cell marker counts predominantly at the dorsal injury site. BrdU cell counts were decreased. Individually and in combination with BrdU, there were reductions in CD68 (monocytes) and Sox2 (immature neural precursors) and increases in Blbp (radial glia) expression. CD68-positive cells showed increased co-staining with iNOS. No differences in the expression of GFAP (glia) and NG2 (oligodendrocytes) or in GFAP cell morphology were found. In conclusion, our work shows that LFS of NRM in subacute SCI influences the proliferation of cell types implicated in inflammation and repair, thus providing mechanistic insight into deep brain stimulation as a neuromodulatory treatment for this devastating pathology.

Keywords: neuromodulation; inflammation; serotonin; neural progenitor cell; deep brain stimulation

1. Introduction

Spinal cord injury (SCI) involves widespread damage of local and distal neuronal networks [1,2]. It is a major cause of disability worldwide, leading to impairments in motor and autonomic function as well as debilitating mechanical allodynia [3–5]. A key difficulty in treating SCI arises from the diversity of cellular processes and physiological functions affected. However, since some degree of functional improvement occurs naturally in the weeks following injury, it is possible that the sequelae of SCI may be overcome to some extent by interventions that enhance endogenous beneficial processes [2,6,7]. Chronic low-frequency electrical stimulation (LFS) of various brain and spinal targets has long been known to influence the perception of chronic pain in select patients [8–10]. However, more recently, LFS of several of these targets and their inputs has received attention for its ability to improve functional outcomes in laboratory and clinical models of SCI [6,11–15]. A critical impediment to the clinical adoption of these treatments is lack of insight into the therapeutic mechanisms involved.

We have previously shown that LFS of the nucleus raphe magnus (NRM) or its primary midbrain afferent, the periaqueductal gray (PAG), improves functional and anatomic recovery from incomplete SCI in rats, while increasing myelination and expression of serotonin- and CGRP-containing axons around the injury site [6,16]. This includes improvements in cutaneous mechanical allodynia [15]. Other sequelae of SCI, such as reduced gastric motility and autonomic dysreflexia, appear to be influenced with LFS of NRM as well [16]. This has led to the proposal that the raphe nuclei of the brainstem, which collectively constitute a system of fibers that diffusely project to most areas of the nervous system, form a key link in a centralized restorative feedback system. The NRM provides a major spinal projection for this system. In support of the generality of this proposed repair model, LFS in the midbrain raphe has been found to improve outcomes in a rat model of traumatic brain injury while LFS in the mouse's NRM ameliorates experimental autoimmune encephalitis (EAE) [14,17].

The mechanisms invoked by brainstem LFS are likely multiple, addressing the multifarious nature of traumatic injuries [2,7,18]. We have previously shown that 2 h of NRM LFS three days after incomplete SCI restores cyclic adenosine monophosphate (cAMP), an intracellular signaling molecule implicated in inflammation and repair, to pre-injury levels [19]. This effect on cAMP is blocked by the non-specific 5-HT$_{7A}$ antagonist pimozide and is accompanied by increases in phosphorylated PKA and CREB, as well as changes in the expression of various genes implicated in inflammation and repair [6,17,19]. We hypothesize that the result is an activation of conserved pathways that blunt secondary injury and enhance restorative processes. To further test this concept, the present study explores whether LFS of NRM initiates changes in the proliferation of immune and neuroglial progenitor cells after incomplete bilateral SCI in the rat.

2. Materials and Methods

2.1. Animal Procedures

This study was conducted under protocols approved by the local Institutional Animal Care and Use Committee. Subjects were young adult female Sprague–Dawley rats (225–250 g), all with injuries. Animals were randomly assigned to two groups: Control ($n = 11$) and LFS ($n = 10$). One rat in the LFS group was lost unexpectedly 12 h after injury. Subgroups were randomly selected for certain markers: eight control and six LFS for the NG2 stain and six control and five LFS for the Blbp/Sox2 stains.

Surgical procedures are described in detail elsewhere [17]. Briefly, under isoflurane anesthesia rats were placed in a stereotaxic holder and cervical laminectomy performed. An Infinite Horizon Impactor (Lexington, KY) produced a midline C5 contusion with a force of 200 kdyn, velocity of 1 m/s, tissue displacement of 0.5 mm, and contact diameter of 2.5 mm. Following impact, the overlying muscle and skin were approximated with nylon sutures. Animals then received a stimulator, which was not activated until 24 h after injury (Figure 1A,B). For controls, stimulators were implanted but never activated. 48 h after injury animals were given a single intraperitoneal dose of bromodeoxyuridine (BrdU, 50–70 μg). Seventy-two hours after injury rats underwent phenobarbital euthanasia and paraformaldehyde perfusion.

2.2. Stimulators

To place stimulators [20], a craniostomy was drilled dorsal to the NRM (2.2 mm caudal, 0 mm lateral, and 1 mm ventral to the interaural line in the horizontal plane). The wireless epoxy-encapsulated stimulator, which measures 12 × 8 × 5 mm and weighs 2 g, was fixed to the skull with screws and dental cement. Two electrodes protrude directly from the capsule: A tungsten microelectrode (cathode) with a resistance of 0.5 megohm at 1 kHz targeted to the NRM, and a stainless-steel wire (anode) attached to a skull screw. Parameters are controlled by a pulsed magnetic field, and it communicates its status via width-modulated infrared pulses received by a custom detector. Status was checked twice daily during the two days animals received LFS. The output consisted of fixed-amplitude 30 μA monopolar pulses with a width of 1.0 ms. The microprocessor cycled between 5 min of 8 Hz stimulation and 5 min of rest during 12 daylight hours [6,14,16,17].

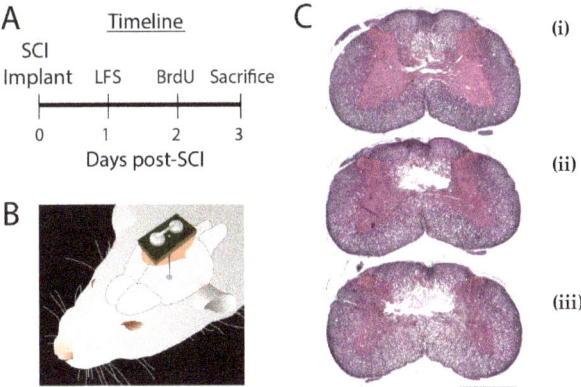

Figure 1. Experimental protocol. (**A**) Experimental timeline. Stimulators were implanted during the same procedure as the C5 contusion but activated one day later in the low-frequency electrical stimulation (LFS) group. (**B**) Schematic illustrating the size and position of the nucleus raphe magnus (NRM) stimulator relative to the rat brain. (**C**) Hematoxylin and eosin-stained sections showing a representative C5 lesion cavity 1 mm rostral to the lesion epicenter (i), at the lesion epicenter (ii), and 1 mm caudal to the lesion epicenter (iii). Scale bar is 1 mm. BrdU, bromodeoxyuridine; LFS, low-frequency stimulation; SCI, spinal cord injury.

2.3. Histological Analysis

Spinal cords were extracted, post-fixed overnight, embedded in paraffin, and sectioned coronally at 12 µm. Slides were deparaffinized with xylene and rehydrated with ethanol and phosphate buffered saline (pH 7.4). Hematoxylin and eosin staining was used to grossly visualize spinal cord lesions (Figure 1C). For immunohistochemical analyses, antigen retrieval was performed in a steam bath with sodium citrate buffer (pH 6.0) for 20 min. Immunostaining was carried out for BrdU, Sox2, Blbp, NG2, GFAP, CD68, iNOS, arginase-1 (arg-1), doublecortin (DCX), NeuN, and APC (Figure 2, Table S1 for antibody details). To reveal BrdU, slides were placed in 4% paraformaldehyde for 20 min, followed by 2 M HCl solution at 37 °C for 30 min prior to application of the primary antibody. Primary antibodies were applied overnight, and secondary antibodies were applied at 1:500 dilution for 2 h. The following markers were co-labeled with BrdU: CD68, GFAP, NG2, Sox2, and Blbp. Other co-labeling combinations were CD68 with Arg1 and iNOS, and NG2 with APC. Staining of nuclei with DAPI was sometimes included. Negative controls using isotype-matched antibodies were examined for each batch of slides.

Cell counts were done by an investigator blinded to animal treatments using epifluorescence microscope-based stereology (Stereo Investigator, Williston, VT). At the level of the lesion, three sections spaced 21 µm apart were used for stereology. For analyses of BrdU, CD68, and GFAP in caudal or rostral tissue, one section 0.75 cm from the lesion epicenter was examined for each location. Separate regional counts were obtained for dorsal white (DWM), ventral white (VWM), and grey matter (GM) after manually tracing these regions at 10×. For each of the three sections, a sampling grid of 225 × 225 µm was placed over each of the three contoured subregions. Within each grid box an area of 75 × 75 µm was selected by the software as the counting frame and cell markers were counted at 60×. The number of counting frames used for each subregion varied between sections but typically ranged from 60 to 90 for DWM, 120 to 180 for GM, and 190 to 270 for VWM.

To examine whether injuries delivered to LFS and control animals differed in intensity, volumetric analyses of lesion cavities was done by tracing sections spaced by 105 µm and aggregating them into a single 3D structure using Callesion software (v1.03) [21].

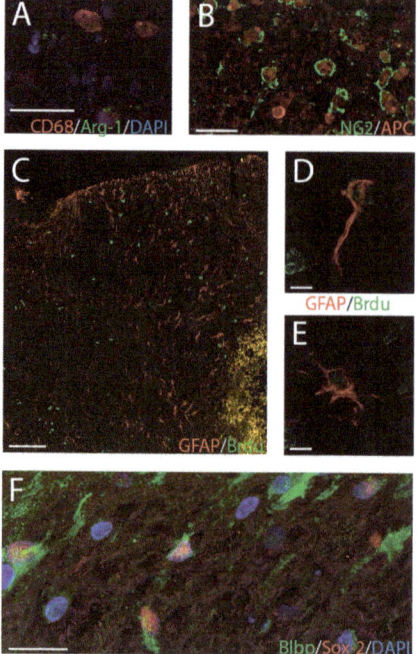

Figure 2. Immunohistochemical analyses. (**A**) Representative immunostain at 60× of an LFS-treated animal showing CD68-positive cells (red) co-labeled with arginase-1 (green) at the lesion. (**B**) Immunostain at 60× of an LFS-treated animal showing cells co-labeled for NG2 (green) and APC (red). (**C**) 10× micrograph through DWM and the lesion cavity showing GFAP (red) and BrdU (green) cells for a control animal. The lesion is seen in the bottom right corner of the image. (**D**) Unipolar GFAP/BrdU cell at 60× for an LFS-treated animal. (**E**) Multipolar GFAP/BrdU cell at 60× for an LFS-treated animal. (**F**) Immunostain at 60× for Blbp (green), Sox2 (red) and DAPI (blue) at the lesion for an LFS-treated animal. The specific immunostains examined and their corresponding colors are shown in the bottom right corner of each panel, except for D and E where this is shown in between the panels. Scale bars are 20 µm for A, B, and F, 100 µm for C, and 10 µm for D and E.

2.4. Statistical Analyses

Quantitative analyses were performed using SPSS (IBM Corporation, Armonk, NY, USA) or spreadsheet calculations, with $p \leq 0.05$ used as the criterion for significance. Comparisons of means, whether for two or three groups, were performed using bootstrap analysis, by resampling data with replacement 1000 times. Multivariate analyses of treatment effects were performed using multinomial logistic regression. In order to have a complete dataset for multivariate analyses, we included only the six LFS and five control rats that were stained for Blbp/Sox2. Stepwise logistic regression analysis was used to define multivariate models that best captured LFS effects.

3. Results

3.1. Did SCI Lesions Differ Between LFS and Control Groups?

Following moderate C5 contusion, flaccid, incomplete quadriplegia was always observed. All animals had shown some recovery of function by the time the animals were euthanized. Histological analysis showed small dorsally located cavities with larger surrounding zones of necrotic tissue. Lesion cavities were generally confined to the DWM and GM, with minimal extension observed into VWM. Volumetric analysis revealed no difference in volume of the lesion cavity between LFS and control animals (0.075 ± 0.016 mm^3 vs. 0.077 ± 0.016 mm^3, $p = 0.38$).

3.2. Were Cellular Effects of LFS Specific to the Injury Site?

BrdU, CD68, and GFAP cell counts were all highest at the lesion as opposed to rostrally or caudally (Table 1, above). The association of LFS with changes in cell counts tended to be greatest at the lesion ($p = 0.10$, three-factor bootstrap). With all spinal cord subregions included, pairwise bootstrap analysis revealed significantly fewer CD68-positive cells ($p = 0.05$), but not BrdU-positive cells ($p = 0.08$), at the lesion in LFS vs. control animals. Significant differences in the counts of these cell markers were not observed for LFS vs. control animals rostral or caudal to the lesion.

Table 1. Effects of LFS of NRM on cell counts for the different spinal cord locations examined.

Marker	Spinal Cord Location					
	Rostral		Lesion		Caudal	
	Control	LFS	Control	LFS	Control	LFS
BrdU	135 ± 14	147 ± 17	587 ± 50	519 ± 49	237 ± 24	209 ± 21
CD68	33 ± 8	34 ± 7	300 ± 39 *	224 ± 28 *	90 ± 21	74 ± 11
GFAP	175 ± 19	206 ± 31	187 ± 29	185 ± 29	114 ± 20	101 ± 23
	DWM		GM		VWM	
	Control	LFS	Control	LFS	Control	LFS
BrdU	105 ± 9	88 ± 11	239 ± 24 *	187 ± 16 *	243 ± 27	234 ± 22
CD68	61 ± 13 *	39 ± 8 *	114 ± 15 *	71 ± 8 *	125 ± 11	114 ± 12
CD68/iNOS	4 ± 2 *	11 ± 4 *	6 ± 2	10 ± 3	6 ± 2	9 ± 3
CD68/Arg-1	5 ± 1	9 ± 3	8 ± 3	13 ± 3	8 ± 2	14 ± 5
GFAP	28 ± 6	28 ± 7	73 ± 11	64 ± 10	86 ± 12	93 ± 12
NG2	81 ± 22 *	149 ± 39 *	46 ± 9	48 ± 10	54 ± 10	55 ± 15
Sox-2	101 ± 16	91 ± 13	155 ± 22 *	78 ± 12 *	128 ± 23 *	81 ± 17 *
Blbp	68 ± 15	102 ± 21	51 ± 8 *	140 ± 25 *	62 ± 15	107 ± 21

Shown are mean (± SE) counts for the various cellular markers examined. The top rows show the counts along the rostro-caudal axis of the spinal cord. The bottom rows show counts at the injury site for the three different spinal cord sub-regions analyzed. *P* values were estimated for individual comparisons using bootstrap analysis and comparisons with $p \leq 0.05$ are marked with *. BrdU, bromodeoxyuridine; DWM, dorsal white matter; LFS, low-frequency stimulation; VWM, ventral white matter.

When cell counts were compared for the different spinal cord subregions at the level of the lesion, their association with LFS was consistently greater at DWM and GM than at VWM (Table 1, below). Given this finding that LFS cellular effects localized predominantly to DWM and GM and the observation that the lesions were confined to DWM and GM histologically, these two subregions were grouped for subsequent analyses (see Table S2 for analyses performed with all spinal cord subregions included).

3.3. Was Immune and Neural Progenitor Cell Expression at the Injury Site Influenced by LFS?

In univariate analysis of the relationship between NRM LFS and the expression of immune and neuroglial progenitor markers, CD68-positive cells were significantly lower in LFS vs. control animals (Figure 3A). CD68-positive cells co-labeled with iNOS were higher in the LFS animals, but CD68 cells co-labeled with arginase-1 did not significantly differ ($p = 0.20$) (Figure 3B,C). GFAP-positive cells typically showed an astrocytic morphology with one or more long processes and with no significant differences in the number of processes between LFS and control animals at the lesion (Figure 3D). In the caudal but not the rostral or lesioned region, the number of GFAP positive cells was increased in the LFS group. NG2-staining cells at the lesion, which typically co-expressed APC suggestive of an oligodendrocyte fate, did not differ between the control and LFS animals (Figure 3E) [7]. Sox2 was predominantly observed in nuclei of ependymal and subependymal cells of the central canal, though positive cells were distributed throughout most areas of the injured cord. The expression of Sox2 was reduced in the LFS animals by about 50%, while Blbp conversely was roughly doubled (Figure 3F,G). Doublecortin-positive cells were not seen in the injured spinal cord.

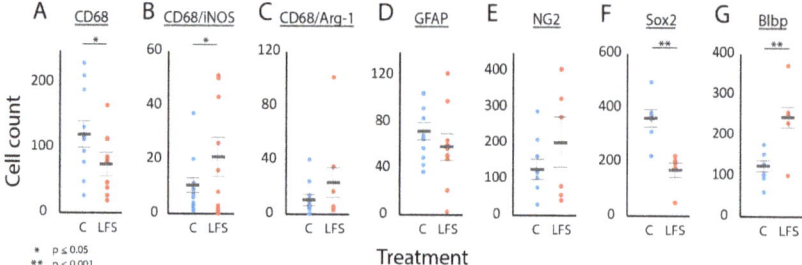

Figure 3. Effects of LFS of NRM on the expression of immune and neuroglial progenitor cell markers at the lesion. Scatter plots comparing cell counts for animals in the control (blue) and LFS (red) groups. Results are shown for CD68 (**A**), CD68/iNOS (**B**), CD68/Arg-1 (**C**), GFAP (**D**), NG2 (**E**), Sox2 (**F**), and Blbp (**G**). Only cell counts from DWM and GM are included. The thick horizontal gray bars show the mean of the counts. The thin horizontal gray bars show standard error. Asterixis above the graphs show statistical significance, if present, which was computed using bootstrap analyses. C, control; LFS, low-frequency stimulation.

Multivariate logistic regression analysis using all immune and neuroglial progenitor cell markers implied a significant LFS-related effect ($F_7 = 20.0$, $p = 0.016$), and stepwise logistic regression gave the following best-fit model for the relation between NRM LFS and changes in cell counts after SCI ($F_3 = 69.2$, $p < 0.001$):

$$\text{NRM LFS} \approx \text{Sox2} + \text{Blbp} + \text{CD68} \tag{1}$$

3.4. Was LFS Associated with Changes in Cellular Proliferation?

The total BrdU count was lower at the lesion for rats treated with LFS of NRM compared to the control animals (Figure 4A–C). At the lesion, BrdU co-labeled with many of the markers examined, including CD68, GFAP, NG2, Blbp, and Sox2, although NeuN did not co-localize with BrdU (Figure 4D–H). CD68 and BrdU co-labeled cells did not achieve statistical significance (Figure 4D) ($p = 0.07$). Univariate analysis indicated a significant relation between LFS and changes in the expression of cells co-localized with Sox2 and BrdU, which were lower in the LFS animals (Figure 4G). Multivariate logistic regression analysis with all regressors found a significant relationship between LFS and the expression of all BrdU co-labeled cells ($F_6 = 7.8$, $p = 0.033$), prominently involving CD68/BrdU ($p = 0.055$) and Blbp/BrdU ($p = 0.056$), although stepwise logistic regression did not produce a model with a significant fit for the effect of LFS on BrdU co-labeled cells.

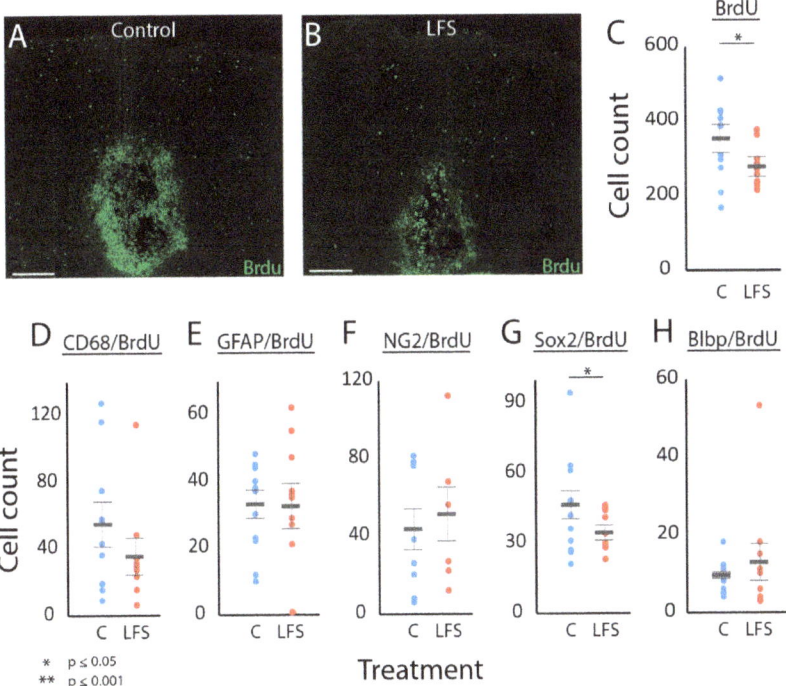

Figure 4. Effects of LFS of NRM on cellular proliferation at the lesion. Representative sections through DWM and GM of LFS-treated (**A**) and control (**B**) animals showing the expression of BrdU-positive cells surrounding the lesion cavity. The scatter plots compare cell counts of BrdU (**C**) and stains co-labeled with BrdU, namely CD68 (**D**), GFAP (**E**), NG2 (**F**), Sox2 (**G**), and Blbp (**H**), for animals in the control (blue) and LFS (red) groups. Only cell counts from DWM and GM are included. The thick horizontal gray bars show the mean of the counts and thin horizontal gray bars show standard error. Asterixis above the graphs denote statistical significance, which was tested for using bootstrap analyses. Scale bar for A and B is 200 µm. C, control; LFS, low-frequency stimulation.

4. Discussion

The present study suggests that treatment of incomplete cervical SCI with two days of LFS in the NRM leads to changes in cellular proliferation in the subacute injury period. Contrary to our expectations, post-injury proliferation was reduced, which we attribute to the treatment reducing inflammation. Other published studies have also shown immune effects of direct or indirect brainstem neuromodulation. LFS of brainstem (PAG, NRM, C1 neurons) or its inputs (vagal nerve, fastigial nucleus) is anti-inflammatory in diverse models of neurologic (Stroke, SCI) and non-neurologic (rheumatoid arthritis, Crohn's disease, sepsis) illness [17,22–24]. Studies of analgesic LFS have also implicated anti-inflammatory mechanisms [25]. In a murine EAE model, our laboratory found that stimulation of NRM prevents disease exacerbation and is associated with reduced spinal cord immune infiltration and cytokine expression [17]. Similarly, vagal nerve stimulation has been shown to reduce disease burden in clinical trials for multiple sclerosis. This neuroinflammatory reflex has been proposed to involve the autonomic nervous system and hippocampal-pituitary-adrenal axis [22–24], but the serotonergic system may be involved as well, as it has been linked to immune control. Serotonin and its receptors are present on numerous cells of the adaptive and innate immune systems and are implicated in microglial activation [26–28].

Although the decreased expression of CD68 is suggestive of anti-inflammatory stimulation effects, the increased co-expression of iNOS and CD68 is inconsistent with this, since iNOS is traditionally a marker of pro-inflammatory macrophages [2,29]. This is likely due to the complex dynamics of macrophage polarization in vivo and our use of the three-day time point. Recent work suggests that sequential activation of both M1 (pro-inflammatory) macrophages, which predominate the first few days after injury, and M2 (anti-inflammatory) macrophages is important for repair after injury [30,31].

Our work also suggests that NRM stimulation influences neuroglial progenitors after SCI. Radial glia, which are increased by LFS in this study, serve as scaffolds for neuronal migration during development and can give rise to new neurons [18,29,30]. Radial glia are associated with repair after injury and they improve functional recovery when injected after SCI in rats [18]. The decrease in Sox2 was unexpected. Sox2 is expressed in immature NPCs of a neuronal lineage. It is co-expressed with Blbp, though Blbp expression is lost earlier in neuronal development. Sox2 maintains the proliferative and developmental potential of NPCs and inhibits the progression from radial glial cell to immature neuron [18,30,31]. We speculate that the depletion of Sox2-positive NPCs here could be caused by increased progression towards a neuronal fate without adequate short-term replenishment, or by the shifting of regenerative resources away from the production of neurons.

The present findings as a whole provide additional support to our hypothesis that the brainstem raphe nuclei are key central links in restorative feedback responses to injury, potentially playing a role in the restorative and analgesic effects of LFS reported previously [6,14,16,17]. Consistent with this model, raphe neurons respond to physiologic correlates of injury, such as pain, low blood pressure, and circulating cytokines, and send diffuse projections to all regions of the neuraxis [26,32]. Although our stimulation protocol precludes elucidation of the precise circuitry, our prior work shows that LFS of NRM leads to synaptic release of serotonin at the SCI site and that therapeutic effects are blocked with a 5-HT$_{7A}$ antagonist, suggesting serotonin may be involved [19]. Serotonin is crucial to the regulation of cell survival during development and is implicated in various protective and trophic processes [26,33,34]. Raphe neurons also secrete several neuropeptides, including galanin, substance P, and thyrotropin-release hormone, that are potentially protective after SCI [32,33]. The relation of NRM LFS to other stimulation targets used for the management of neurotrauma (vagal nerve, periaqueductal grey, spinal cord), for which the modulation of autonomic function is a commonly proposed mechanism, is unclear [6,8,14,16,17,19,35]. However, given the established reciprocal connections between these targets, it is likely that diverse overlapping processes are elicited with each stimulation target [14,26,32].

This study also gives credence to prior clinical and laboratory studies that suggest a potential role for neuromodulatory therapies in the management of SCI and its sequelae [6,11–13,15]. Although the elucidation of precise mechanisms of action of NRM LFS was beyond the scope of this work, the implication of cell markers known to be involved in inflammation and repair is intriguing, since these processes have been commonly targeted before in attempts to restore function following SCI [13,25,36]. Neuromodulatory treatments of SCI, in general, would be welcome by the clinical community, since deep brain and spinal cord stimulation and the associated devices are already accepted as safe and effective for various other neurologic indications, reducing potential regulatory hurdles to their approval for SCI [10].

One limitation of this study was the analysis of a single time point at three days. This time point was used because it allowed us to obtain a broad snapshot of protective and restorative processes at a critical post-injury period when these processes are often at their peak [2,7]. Additionally, our prior studies found molecular, genetic, and behavioral effects of NRM LFS on injured spinal cord to be maximal when applied during this post-injury period. Another limitation was lack of behavioral data, which was not included due to the short post-injury survival period used here and because our prior work has shown that the therapeutic effect of NRM LFS reveals itself over longer experimental periods [6,16,17]. Another limitation is that, because this was a correlational study, the cellular effects, if any, that would contribute to or result from the improvements in functional recovery are unclear.

5. Conclusions

A satisfactory treatment for pain and other signs of incomplete SCI does not yet exist but will ultimately require not only inhibiting detrimental secondary processes, such as edema and inflammation, but also recruiting cells that support regeneration. The targeting of brainstem centers that have multiple beneficial effects is a potential means towards accomplishing these goals, with the major strategic advantage that a single existing clinical tool is used. Prior to clinical application of this therapy, however, it will be important to better define the treatment's mechanisms and their influence on recovery, for both the NRM and for various other promising stimulation targets. This approach can not only provide hope for improving the devastating outcomes associated with SCI but also improve our basic understanding of the brain's central responses to SCI and their role in coordinating the necessarily incomplete process of natural recovery.

Supplementary Materials: The following are available online at http://www.mdpi.com/2076-3425/9/6/124/s1, Table S1: List of antibodies and concentrations used; Supplemental; Table S2: Univariate and multivariate regression analyses with all three spinal cord subregions included in analyses.

Author Contributions: Conceptualization, W.J.J., M.M.C.-G., I.D.H.; methodology, W.J.J., M.M.C.-G. and I.D.H.; validation, W.J.J., L.D.; formal analysis, W.J.J., I.D.H.; investigation, S.S.S., L.D., A.V., M.M.C.-G.; resources, I.D.H.; data curation, L.D.; writing—original draft preparation, W.J.J., I.D.H.; writing—review and editing, W.J.J., M.M.C.-G., I.D.H.; visualization, W.J.J.; supervision, W.J.J.; project administration, W.J.J., I.D.H.; funding acquisition, I.D.H.

Funding: This work was supported by funding from The Robert J. Kleberg, Jr. and Helen C. Kleberg Foundation, The Craig H. Neilsen Foundation, and the Miami Project to Cure Paralysis.

Acknowledgments: The authors thank Ross Bullock and Shyam Gajavelli for their technical assistance.

Conflicts of Interest: The authors declare no conflict of interest.

References

1. Chen, L.M.; Mishra, A.; Yang, P.F.; Wang, F.; Gore, J.C. Injury alters intrinsic functional connectivity within the primate spinal cord. *Proc. Natl. Acad. Sci. USA* **2015**, *112*, 5991–5996. [CrossRef]
2. David, S.; Kroner, A. Repertoire of microglial and macrophage responses after spinal cord injury. *Nat. Rev. Neurosci.* **2011**, *12*, 388–399. [CrossRef] [PubMed]
3. Attal, N.; Fermanian, C.; Fermanian, J.; Lanteri-Minet, M.; Alchaar, H.; Bouhassira, D. Neuropathic pain: Are there distinct subtypes depending on the aetiology or anatomical lesion? *Pain* **2008**, *138*, 343–353. [CrossRef] [PubMed]
4. Gooch, C.L.; Pracht, E.; Borenstein, A.R. The burden of neurological disease in the United States: A summary report and call to action. *Ann. Neurol.* **2017**, *81*, 479–484. [CrossRef] [PubMed]
5. Martin, B.I.; Deyo, R.A.; Mirza, S.K.; Turner, J.A.; Comstock, B.A.; Hollingworth, W.; Sullivan, S.D. Expenditures and health status among adults with back and neck problems. *JAMA* **2008**, *299*, 656–664. [CrossRef]
6. Hentall, I.D.; Gonzalez, M.M. Promotion of recovery from thoracic spinal cord contusion in rats by stimulation of medullary raphe or its midbrain input. *Neurorehabil. Neural Repair* **2012**, *26*, 374–384. [CrossRef] [PubMed]
7. Mao, Y.; Mathews, K.; Gorrie, C.A. Temporal Response of Endogenous Neural Progenitor Cells Following Injury to the Adult Rat Spinal Cord. *Front. Cell Neurosci.* **2016**, *10*, 58. [CrossRef] [PubMed]
8. Jermakowicz, W.J.; Hentall, I.D.; Jagid, J.R.; Luca, C.C.; Adcock, J.; Martinez-Arizala, A.; Widerstrom-Noga, E. Deep Brain Stimulation Improves the Symptoms and Sensory Signs of Persistent Central Neuropathic Pain from Spinal Cord Injury: A Case Report. *Front. Hum. Neurosci.* **2017**, *11*, 177. [CrossRef]
9. Keay, K.A.; Bandler, R. Periaqueductal Gray. In *The Rat Nervous System*, 4th ed.; Elsevier: Waltham, MA, USA, 2015.
10. Pereira, E.A.; Aziz, T.Z. Neuropathic pain and deep brain stimulation. *Neurotherapeutics* **2014**, *11*, 496–507. [CrossRef]
11. Vasudeva, V.S.; Abd-El-Barr, M.; Chi, J. Lumbosacral spinal cord epidural stimulation enables recovery of voluntary movement after complete motor spinal cord injury. *Neurosurgery* **2014**, *75*, N14–N15. [CrossRef]

12. McPherson, J.G.; Miller, R.R.; Perlmutter, S.I. Targeted, activity-dependent spinal stimulation produces long-lasting motor recovery in chronic cervical spinal cord injury. *Proc. Natl. Acad. Sci. USA* **2015**, *112*, 12193–12198. [CrossRef] [PubMed]
13. Li, Q.; Brus-Ramer, M.; Martin, J.H.; McDonald, J.W. Electrical stimulation of the medullary pyramid promotes proliferation and differentiation of oligodendrocyte progenitor cells in the corticospinal tract of the adult rat. *Neurosci. Lett.* **2010**, *479*, 128–133. [CrossRef] [PubMed]
14. Carballosa Gonzalez, M.M.; Blaya, M.O.; Alonso, O.F.; Bramlett, H.M.; Hentall, I.D. Midbrain raphe stimulation improves behavioral and anatomical recovery from fluid-percussion brain injury. *J. Neurotrauma* **2013**, *30*, 119–130. [CrossRef]
15. Hentall, I.D.; Burns, S.B. Restorative effects of stimulating medullary raphe after spinal cord injury. *J. Rehabil. Res. Dev.* **2009**, *46*, 109–122. [CrossRef]
16. Vitores, A.A.; Sloley, S.S.; Martinez, C.; Carballosa-Gautam, M.M.; Hentall, I.D. Some Autonomic Deficits of Acute or Chronic Cervical Spinal Contusion Reversed by Interim Brainstem Stimulation. *J. Neurotrauma* **2018**, *35*, 560–572. [CrossRef]
17. Madsen, P.M.; Sloley, S.S.; Vitores, A.A.; Carballosa-Gautam, M.M.; Brambilla, R.; Hentall, I.D. Prolonged stimulation of a brainstem raphe region attenuates experimental autoimmune encephalomyelitis. *Neuroscience* **2017**, *346*, 395–402. [CrossRef]
18. Chang, Y.W.; Goff, L.A.; Li, H.; Kane-Goldsmith, N.; Tzatzalos, E.; Hart, R.P.; Young, W.; Grumet, M. Rapid induction of genes associated with tissue protection and neural development in contused adult spinal cord after radial glial cell transplantation. *J. Neurotrauma* **2009**, *26*, 979–993. [CrossRef]
19. Carballosa-Gonzalez, M.M.; Vitores, A.; Hentall, I.D. Hindbrain raphe stimulation boosts cyclic adenosine monophosphate and signaling proteins in the injured spinal cord. *Brain Res.* **2014**, *1543*, 165–172. [CrossRef]
20. Hentall, I.D. A long-lasting wireless stimulator for small mammals. *Front. Neuroengin.* **2013**, *6*, 8. [CrossRef] [PubMed]
21. Park, H.J.; Machado, A.G.; Cooperrider, J.; Truong-Furmaga, H.; Johnson, M.; Krishna, V.; Chen, Z.; Gale, J.T. Semi-automated method for estimating lesion volumes. *J. Neurosci. Methods* **2013**, *213*, 76–83. [CrossRef] [PubMed]
22. Tang, W.; Dong, W.; Xie, P.; Cheng, P.; Bai, S.; Ren, Y.; Wang, G.; Chen, X.; Cui, C.; Zhuang, Y.; et al. The Effect of Pre-Condition Cerebella Fastigial Nucleus Electrical Stimulation within and beyond the Time Window of Thrombolytic on Ischemic Stroke in the Rats. *PLoS ONE* **2015**, *10*, e0128447. [CrossRef]
23. Rasmussen, S.E.; Pfeiffer-Jensen, M.; Drewes, A.M.; Farmer, A.D.; Deleuran, B.W.; Stengaard-Pedersen, K.; Brock, B.; Brock, C. Vagal influences in rheumatoid arthritis. *Scand. J. Rheumatol.* **2018**, *47*, 1–11. [CrossRef]
24. Abe, C.; Inoue, T.; Inglis, M.A.; Viar, K.E.; Huang, L.; Ye, H.; Rosin, D.L.; Stornetta, R.L.; Okusa, M.D.; Guyenet, P.G. C1 neurons mediate a stress-induced anti-inflammatory reflex in mice. *Nat. Neurosci.* **2017**, *20*, 700–707. [CrossRef]
25. Kiguchi, N.; Kobayashi, D.; Saika, F.; Matsuzaki, S.; Kishioka, S. Pharmacological Regulation of Neuropathic Pain Driven by Inflammatory Macrophages. *Int. J. Mol. Sci.* **2017**, *18*, 2296. [CrossRef]
26. Baganz, N.L.; Blakely, R.D. A dialogue between the immune system and brain, spoken in the language of serotonin. *ACS Chem. Neurosci.* **2013**, *4*, 48–63. [CrossRef]
27. Jiang, X.; Wang, J.; Luo, T.; Li, Q. Impaired hypothalamic-pituitary-adrenal axis and its feedback regulation in serotonin transporter knockout mice. *Psychoneuroendocrinology* **2009**, *34*, 317–331. [CrossRef] [PubMed]
28. Krabbe, G.; Matyash, V.; Pannasch, U.; Mamer, L.; Boddeke, H.W.; Kettenmann, H. Activation of serotonin receptors promotes microglial injury-induced motility but attenuates phagocytic activity. *Brain Behav. Immun.* **2012**, *26*, 419–428. [CrossRef]
29. Goldshmit, Y.; Frisca, F.; Pinto, A.R.; Pebay, A.; Tang, J.K.; Siegel, A.L.; Kaslin, J.; Currie, P.D. Fgf2 improves functional recovery-decreasing gliosis and increasing radial glia and neural progenitor cells after spinal cord injury. *Brain Behav.* **2014**, *4*, 187–200. [CrossRef]
30. Gomez-Lopez, S.; Wiskow, O.; Favaro, R.; Nicolis, S.K.; Price, D.J.; Pollard, S.M.; Smith, A. Sox2 and Pax6 maintain the proliferative and developmental potential of gliogenic neural stem cells In vitro. *Glia* **2011**, *59*, 1588–1599. [CrossRef]

31. Li, T.; Peng, M.; Yang, Z.; Zhou, X.; Deng, Y.; Jiang, C.; Xiao, M.; Wang, J. 3D-printed IFN-gamma-loading calcium silicate-beta-tricalcium phosphate scaffold sequentially activates M1 and M2 polarization of macrophages to promote vascularization of tissue engineering bone. *Acta Biomater* **2018**, *71*, 96–107. [CrossRef] [PubMed]
32. Calizo, L.H.; Akanwa, A.; Ma, X.; Pan, Y.Z.; Lemos, J.C.; Craige, C.; Heemstra, L.A.; Beck, S.G. Raphe serotonin neurons are not homogenous: Electrophysiological, morphological and neurochemical evidence. *Neuropharmacology* **2011**, *61*, 524–543. [CrossRef] [PubMed]
33. Choi, M.; Son, H. Effects of serotonin on erythropoietin expression in mouse hippocampus. *Exp. Neurobiol.* **2013**, *22*, 45–50. [CrossRef]
34. Arnold, S.A.; Hagg, T. Serotonin 1A receptor agonist increases species- and region-selective adult CNS proliferation, but not through CNTF. *Neuropharmacology* **2012**, *63*, 1238–1247. [CrossRef]
35. Ievins, A.; Moritz, C.T. Therapeutic Stimulation for Restoration of Function After Spinal Cord Injury. *Physiology (Bethesda)* **2017**, *32*, 391–398. [CrossRef] [PubMed]
36. Arnold, S.A.; Hagg, T. Anti-inflammatory treatments during the chronic phase of spinal cord injury improve locomotor function in adult mice. *J. Neurotrauma* **2011**, *28*, 1995–2002. [CrossRef]

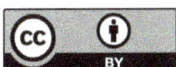

© 2019 by the authors. Licensee MDPI, Basel, Switzerland. This article is an open access article distributed under the terms and conditions of the Creative Commons Attribution (CC BY) license (http://creativecommons.org/licenses/by/4.0/).

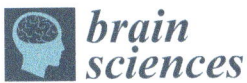

Case Report

Antiplatelet Versus Anticoagulation for Asymptomatic Patients with Vertebral Artery Injury During Anterior Cervical Surgery—Two Case Reports and Review of Literature

Michael Hall [1], David Cheng [2], Wayne Cheng [2] and Olumide Danisa [2],*

1. UCR School of Medicine, Riverside, CA 92507, USA; Mhall015@medsch.ucr.edu
2. Loma Linda Medical Center, Loma Linda, CA 92354, USA; Davidwaynecheng@gmail.com (D.C.); Spinesurgeon1995@gmail.com (W.C.)
* Correspondence: Odanisa@llu.edu

Received: 22 October 2019; Accepted: 22 November 2019; Published: 28 November 2019

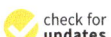

Abstract: Vertebral Artery Injury (VAI) while performing cervical spinal reconstruction surgery is rare, but it can lead to catastrophic events. Treatment for this injury with regard to antiplatelet versus anticoagulation therapy is controversial. The purpose of this report is to discuss two cases of VAI that occurred during the performance of cervical reconstruction surgery and provide a guideline based on a literature review about whether to use anticoagulant or antiplatelet therapy for treatment of asymptomatic VAI. In case 1, iatrogenic injury occurred to the left C5 vertebral artery (VA) during high speed burr removal of an osteophyte on the left C5/6 uncovertebral joint, resulting in VAI. This patient was treated with Heparin resulting in respiratory complication. Case 2 encountered VAI while using the kerrison rongeur to perform a right sided C5/6 foraminotomy. Antiplatelet therapy was administered. Fourteen publications relevant to Antiplatelet versus Anticoagulation treatment were reviewed. Anticoagulation has similar results to antiplatelet therapy. Studies are limited; there were no common guidelines or parameters concerning the utilization of Antiplatelets versus Anticoagulants. Anticoagulation achieved similar results as Antiplatelet therapy; based on the limited relevant data, the superiority of one treatment over the other cannot be concluded in VAI after cervical spinal reconstruction surgery.

Keywords: antiplatelets; anticoagulation; vertebral artery injury; cervical surgery

1. Introduction

Vertebral Artery Injury (VAI) can be a devastating event due to causing the following—arterial dissection, hematoma formation, aneurysm or vascular occlusion. This in turn can result in fatal ischemic injury or potentially permanent neurological impairment. Unilateral damage to the vertebral artery (VA), fortunately, is rarely deadly due to the contribution of collateral circulation (contralateral VA and the Circle of Willis) [1]. Injury to this artery is common in cervical blunt trauma [2]. During surgical procedures, such as an anterior corpectomy or anterior cervical fusion, the VA remains vulnerable due to its unique anatomical location within the C2–C6 transverse foramina. Various clinical syndromes can manifest from this injury, such as lateral medullary syndrome (Wallenberg Syndrome) [3].

Treatment options for VAI are—observation, anticoagulation or antiplatelet therapy. No preferred method has been proven to be superior [4]. The controversy of anticoagulation versus antiplatelet therapy is a topic of interest in the field of spine surgery. Literature concerning this controversy is limited. In our case presentations, we decided to treat with anticoagulation therapy in one patient, and with antiplatelet therapy in the other.

2. Materials and Methods

We report two cases of VAI after anterior cervical surgery at our institution from 2015 to 2017. The radiographic features, presenting symptoms, clinical characteristics, type of management and outcomes of the patients were all studied. A literature review was also conducted to evaluate the current management and treatment of asymptomatic VAI—observation, anticoagulation or antiplatelet therapy.

3. Results

3.1. Case Reports

3.1.1. Case Illustration 1

Patient is a 78 year-old male presenting with history of cervical myelopathy—frequent falls over the past 12 months, difficulty with bowel and bladder control and complaints of diminished dexterity of the hands.

3.1.2. Imaging

Plain X-rays revealed large anterior osteophytes most prominent from C4–C7 with severe spondylosis. MRI images show spinal cord compression from C4–C7 and myelomalacia at C5–C6, retrolisthesis at C4–C5, and severe multilevel disk degeneration (Figure 1).

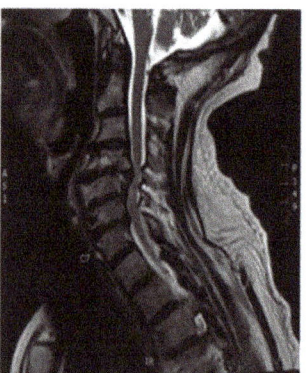

Figure 1. Pre-op Sagittal Magnetic Resonance Image (MRI) (Cervical Spine).

3.1.3. Surgical Plan

Stage 1—anterior corpectomy at C5, fibula structural allograft, anterior discectomy at C6–C7 and a C4–C7 anterior fusion instrumentation. Stage 2—posterior C4 to C7 posterior decompressive laminectomies, fusion, instrumentation and bone graft.

3.1.4. Surgical Complication

During Stage I surgery, pulsatile bleeding was encountered when using a high speed burr to remove an osteophyte on the left of C5/6 uncovertebral joint vertebral body. Bone wax was applied to regain hemodynamic control. Four hundred ml of blood was lost but the remainder of the surgery was uneventful.

The patient was asymptomatic immediately post-op. Computed tomography (CT) angiography showed anterolateral bony defect at C5 (Figure 2). The study also revealed 50% focal narrowing of the left VA at C5; consistent with focal thrombus versus external compression possibly due to bone wax (Figure 3). The study confirmed acceptable cervical alignment, operative decompression, and hardware placement.

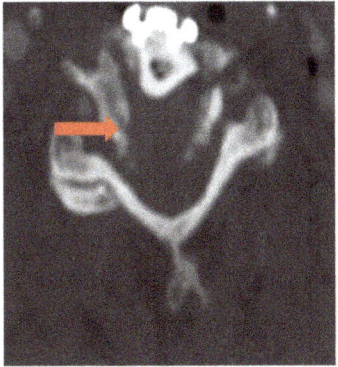

Figure 2. Computed tomography (CT) Scan (arrow denoting bony defect C5).

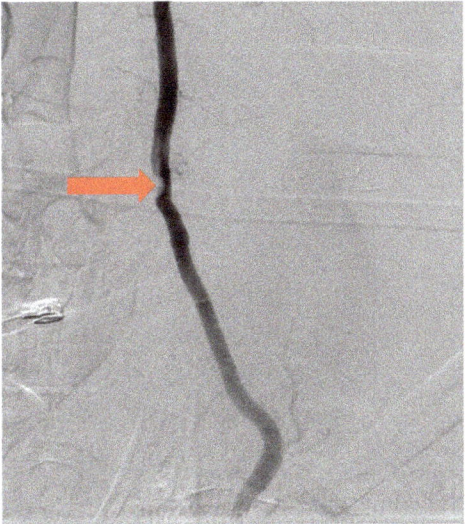

Figure 3. Angiogram (arrow denoting filling defect).

3.1.5. Case Illustration 1

The patient was admitted to the intensive care unit and Mean Arterial Pressures (MAPs) were maintained at 90 mmHg, and he was fully anticoagulated with a heparin drip. He, however, developed significant airway edema and respiratory distress within 24 h after anticoagulation and hypertensive therapy. The patient thus required emergent intubation and subsequent operative hematoma evacuation. Lateral radiograph 1-year post operation shows C4–C7 fusion hardware and resolution of hemodynamic instability (Figure 4).

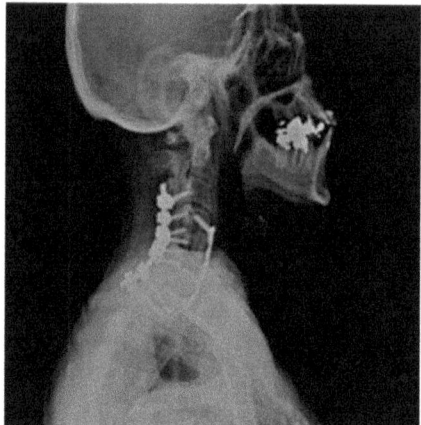

Figure 4. Lateral Radiograph Post Op 1 Year.

3.1.6. Case Illustration 2

The patient is a 57 year-old female with a past medical history (PMH) positive for a pacemaker and an embolic cerebral vascular event (CVA) at age 50. She presented with a 9-month history of cervical radiculopathy manifested by severe neck pain, right shoulder and arm pain, along with mild weakness in the right biceps. Sensory deficits noted in the C5 and C6 dermatomes. She had failed conservative management (physical therapy, chiropractic manipulation, acupuncture) and cervical epidural.

3.1.7. Imaging

Plain radiograph showed multi-level cervical spondylosis. CT myelogram of the cervical spine from an outside institution demonstrated cervical stenosis, worst at the C4/5 and C5/6 levels (Figure 5). Magnetic Resonance Imaging (MRI) was unable to be performed due to lack of insurance authorization.

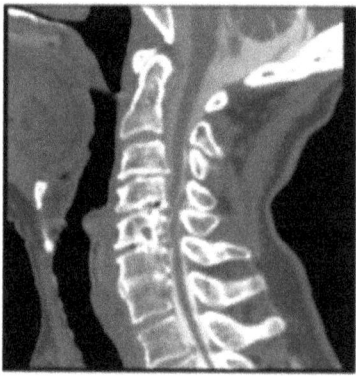

Figure 5. CT myelogram.

3.1.8. Surgical Plan

C4/5 and C5/6 anterior cervical discectomy and fusion (ACDF) with central and foraminal decompressions at corresponding levels.

3.1.9. Surgical Complication

During the right sided foraminotomy at C5/6, brisk bleeding was noted while using a kerrison rongeur to remove the medial uncovertebral joint. Hemostatic agents and cottonoids were used in unison to control the bleeding. A total of 500 mL of blood was lost. Despite a brief decrease in blood pressure, hemodynamics was stabilized with rapid crystalloid and albumin infusion. Neuromonitoring signals (transcranial MEPs and SSEPs) were stable throughout. The surgery was completed—interbody allograft cages placed, and 2-level plate implanted from C4–C6.

3.2. Case Illustration 2

The patient was extubated and taken to the recovery room. Her blood pressure and pulse rate were within normal range. Her neurologic exam was intact with regard to mentation, coordination and motor function. Sensory deficits were unchanged from pre-operative exam. She was taken to the angiography suite and this revealed occlusion of the right VA (Figure 6). She had a contrast brain CT 48 h later, and no evidence of ischemia or infarct was noted. She subsequently was started on Aspirin (ASA) therapy on post-op day # 3. Serial exams throughout her 5-day hospitalization remained unchanged except for improvement in pre-operative sensory deficit. Follow up angiogram 6 months later showed recanalization of right VA (Figure 7).

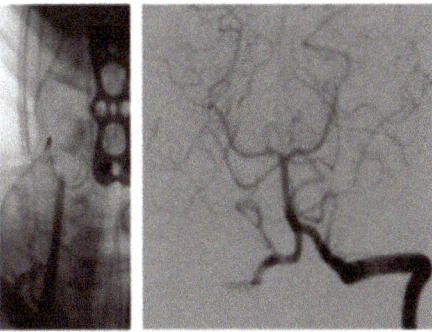

Figure 6. Angiogram post-op.

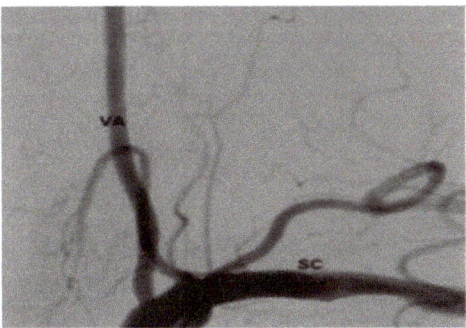

Figure 7. Angiogram 6 months post-op.

4. Discussion

Case 1 details a case of respiratory distress and airway complications due to postoperative anticoagulant therapy which necessitated emergent intubation and hematoma evacuation. In this case, we decided to treat with anticoagulant (Heparin) therapy after asymptomatic operative VAI.

According to the literature, anticoagulant management post VAI has traditionally led to hemodynamic stabilization [5–7].

Case 2 also encountered VAI, this time while using the kerrison rongeur to perform a right sided C5/6 foraminotomy. We decided to treat this patient with delayed antiplatelet therapy due to a lack of postoperative neurologic deficits.

Lunardini et al. [8] published a cervical spine research society (CSRS) cross-sectional study where members were surveyed and the incidence of VAI was reported as 0.07% (111/163,324) of cervical surgeries. The specific surgical procedures were extrapolated—posterior instrumentation of the cervical spine (32.4%), anterior cervical corpectomy (23.4%), and posterior cervical exposure (11.7%), anterior discectomy (9%). Outcomes of the VAI showed no permanent neurologic sequelae in 90% of patients, permanent neurologic sequelae in 5.5%, and death in 4%. It was also concluded that less experienced surgeons (performed fewer than 300 cervical lifetime cases) had a fivefold increased risk of causing an iatrogenic VAI. Guan et al. [9] performed a systematic review of 25 papers reporting VAI injury in 54 patients after anterior cervical surgery for the following conditions: degenerative disease (64%), tumor (14%), and trauma (9%). They concluded that preoperative evaluation (including angiography) and real time radiographic guidance reduced VAI risk. They also cautioned against the use of tamponade as definitive treatment since there is a 48% pseudoaneurysm risk.

In our case series, neither patient was asymptomatic after sustaining iatrogenic VAI. In both cases, we did not feel the need for endovascular repair. The issue, then is how to manage the complications. The use of antiplatelet vs anticoagulation therapy for management of VAI remains a controversial topic, there is no substantive literature displaying superiority of a particular pharmacologic modality.

5. Literature Review

5.1. Anticoagulation Therapy

General guidelines of asymptomatic VAI management involve observation, anticoagulation or antiplatelet modalities [10]. A case series by Schellinger et al. [11] evaluated 4 patients with VAI. Two (50%) patients suffered ischemic mortality from observation without therapy while 1 (25%) symptomatic patient received Heparin leading to resolution of symptoms and 1 (25%) symptomatic patient received no therapy resulting in symptom resolution [11].

In another case series, Willis et al. [12] evaluated 12 asymptomatic patients with VAI. Nine of 12 (75%) patients suffered vertebral artery occlusion (VAO) only to be treated with observation, none suffered ischemic complications. Three of the 12 (25%) patients had evidence of pseudoaneurysm or dissection successfully treated with systemic Heparin [12].

Biffl et al. [5] found that VAI patients treated with systemic Heparin were associated with improved neurological outcomes and decreased incidence of neurological deterioration from onset injury to discharge. Of the 16 VAI patients treated with systemic heparin within the study, 2 (13%) improved, only 4 (25%) increased to higher injury grade and 10 (63%) remained unchanged [5].

5.2. Antiplatelet Therapy

Conversely, in another study by Colella et al. [13], 9 patients with mural carotid injury were treated with antiplatelet therapy resulting in 8 (88%) patients recovering neurologically without deficits. Jang et al. [7] conducted a study to evaluate the management of asymptomatic VAO in 8 patients needing cervical fracture surgery. Five of 8 (62%) patients were treated by observation alone while 2 of 8 (25%) patients were treated with aspirin post-operatively, all making a complete recovery without heparin use [7].

5.3. Anticoagulation vs. Antiplatelet Therapy

A randomized control trial by the Cervical Artery in Dissection Stroke Study(CADISS) investigators [14] assessed the efficacy of antiplatelets versus anticoagulants in the treatment of extracranial VA dissection. No statistical difference between the two treatments was appreciated ($p = 0.2$). Of the 126 patients treated with antiplatelet modalities, 3 (2%) experienced death or stroke while 1 patient experienced stroke of the 124 treated with anticoagulant modalities (odds ratio [OR] 0.335, 95% CI 0.006–4.233; $p = 0.63$) [14].

6. Conclusions

The overall risk of VAI in cervical surgery is low. The majority of VAI have no permanent neurologic impairment, yet this injury serves as a cautionary tale. At our institution, we are currently considering routine preoperative angiography for high risk cases such as anterior cervical corpectomy. We are also starting to implement intraoperative navigation for such cases. First line medical management for asymptomatic VAI includes—observation, anticoagulation and antiplatelet therapy. The therapeutic management of VAI regarding anticoagulation versus antiplatelet modalities are controversial. Conflicting evidence based on the literature makes establishing a preferred method in the management of asymptomatic VAI difficult. The definitive establishment of anticoagulation over antiplatelet therapy or vice versa as the superior method in asymptomatic VAI treatment, is inconclusive. Due to the increased variability in outcomes of asymptomatic VAI treatment; the controversy between antiplatelet and anticoagulation therapy remains.

Author Contributions: Conceptualization, O.D., W.C., M.H., and D.C.; Methodology, M.H., D.C., W.C., and O.D.; Software, D.C. and M.H.; Validation, O.D. and W.C.; Formal Analysis, O.D., W.C., M.H., and D.C.; Investigation, O.D., W.C., M.H., and D.C.; Resources, D.C. and M.H.; Data Curation, O.D. and W.C.; Writing—Original Draft Preparation, M.H. and D.C.; Writing—Review & Editing, M.H., D.C., W.C., and O.D.; Visualization, O.D., W.C., M.H., and D.C.; Supervision, O.D. and W.C.; Project Administration, O.D. and W.C.

Funding: This research received no external funding.

Conflicts of Interest: The authors declare no conflict of interest.

References

1. Markus, H.S.; Levi, C.; King, A.; Madigan, J.; Norris, J. Antiplatelet treatment compared with anticoagulation treatment for cervical artery dissection (CADISS): A randomized trial. *Lancet Neurol.* **2015**, *14*, 361–367. [CrossRef] [PubMed]
2. Griffin, R.L.; Falatko, S.R.; Aslibekyan, S.; Strickland, V.; Harrigan, M.R. Aspirin for primary prevention of stroke in traumatic cerebrovascular injury: Association with increased risk of transfusion. *J. Neurosurg.* **2018**, *130*, 1520–1527. [CrossRef] [PubMed]
3. Daou, B.; Hammer, C.; Mouchtouris, N.; Starke, R.M.; Koduri, S.; Yang, S.; Jabbour, P.; Rosenwasser, R.; Tjoumakaris, S. Anticoagulation vs Antiplatelet Treatment in Patients with Carotid and Vertebral Artery Dissection: A Study of 370 Patients and Literature Review. *Neurosurgery* **2017**, *80*, 368–379. [CrossRef] [PubMed]
4. Nassenstein, I.; Krämer, S.C.; Niederstadt, T.; Stehling, C.; Dittrich, R.; Kuhlenbäumer, G.; Ringelstein, E.B.; Heindel, W.; Bachmann, R. Incidence of cerebral ischemia in patients with suspected cervical artery dissection: First results of a prospective study. *Rofo* **2005**, *177*, 1532–1539. [CrossRef] [PubMed]
5. Biffl, W.L.; Moore, E.E.; Elliott, J.P.; Ray, C.; Offner, P.J.; Franciose, R.J.; Brega, K.E.; Burch, J.M. The devastating potential of blunt vertebral arterial injuries. *Ann. Surg.* **2000**, *231*, 672–681. [CrossRef] [PubMed]
6. Fassett, D.R.; Dailey, A.T.; Vaccaro, A.R. Vertebral artery injuries associated with cervical spine injuries: A review of the literature. *Clin. Spine Surg.* **2008**, *21*, 252–258. [CrossRef] [PubMed]
7. Jang, D.; Kim, C.; Lee, S.J.; Kim, J. Delayed Brain Infarction due to Bilateral Vertebral Artery Occlusion Which Occurred 5 Days after Cervical Trauma. *J. Korean Neurosurg. Soc.* **2014**, *56*, 141–145. [CrossRef] [PubMed]
8. Lunardini, D.J.; Eskander, M.S.; Even, J.L.; Dunlap, J.T.; Chen, A.F.; Lee, J.Y.; Ward, T.W.; Kang, J.D.; Donaldson, W.F. Vertebral artery injuries in cervical spine surgery. *Spine J.* **2014**, *14*, 1520–1525. [CrossRef] [PubMed]
9. Guan, Q.; Chen, L.; Long, Y.; Xiang, Z. Iatrogenic Vertebral Artery Injury during Anterior Cervical Spine Surgery: A Systematic Review. *World Neurosurg.* **2017**, *106*, 715–722. [CrossRef] [PubMed]

10. Simon, L.V.; Mohseni, M. *Vertebral Artery Injury, Treasure Island (FL)*; StatPearls Publishing: Petersburg, FL, USA, 2018.
11. Schellinger, P.D.; Schwab, S.; Krieger, D.; Fiebach, J.B.; Steiner, T.; Hund, E.F.; Hacke, W.; Meinck, H.M. Masking of vertebral artery dissection by severe trauma to the cervical spine. *Spine* **2001**, *26*, 314–319. [CrossRef] [PubMed]
12. Willis, B.K.; Greiner, F.; Orrison, W.W.; Benzel, E.C. The incidence of vertebral artery injury after midcervical spine fracture or subluxation. *Neurosurgery* **1994**, *34*, 435–442. [CrossRef] [PubMed]
13. Colella, J.J.; Diamond, D.L. Blunt Carotid Injury: Reassessing the role of anticoagulation. *Am. J. Surg.* **1996**, *62*, 212–217.
14. Caplan, L.R. Antiplatelets vs. anticoagulation for dissection: CADISS nonrandomized arm and meta-analysis. *Neurology* **2013**, *80*, 970–971. [CrossRef] [PubMed]

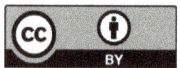

© 2019 by the authors. Licensee MDPI, Basel, Switzerland. This article is an open access article distributed under the terms and conditions of the Creative Commons Attribution (CC BY) license (http://creativecommons.org/licenses/by/4.0/).

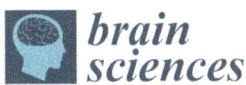

Perspective

Disseminated Coccidioidomycosis to the Spine—Case Series and Review of Literature

Dinesh Ramanathan, Nikhil Sahasrabudhe and Esther Kim *

Loma Linda University Medical Center, Loma Linda, CA 92354, USA
* Correspondence: Estkim@llu.edu

Received: 31 May 2019; Accepted: 5 July 2019; Published: 7 July 2019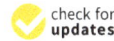

Abstract: Coccidioidomycosis is a fungal infectious disease caused by the *Coccidioides* species endemic to Southwestern United States. Symptomatic patients typically present as community-acquired pneumonia. Uncommonly, in about 1% of infections, hematogenous extra pulmonary systemic dissemination involving skin, musculoskeletal system, and meninges occur. Disseminated spinal infection is treated with antifungal drugs and/or surgical treatment. A retrospective review of medical records at our institution was done between January 2009 to December 2018 and we present three cases of spinal coccidioidomycosis and review the current literature. Disseminated coccidioidomycosis can lead to spondylitis that can present as discitis or a localized spinal or paraspinal abscess. Spinal coccidioidomycosis is typically managed with antifungal treatments but can include surgical treatment in the setting poor response to medical therapy, intractable pain, presence of neurological deficits due to compression, or structural spinal instability.

Keywords: Coccidioidomycosis; spinal infection; spinal pain

1. Introduction

Coccidiomycosis is a fungal infectious disease caused by the *Coccidioides* species endemic to Southwestern United States. Also known as Valley fever, it is caused by *Coccidioides immitis* or *Coccidioides posadasii*. These organisms survive well in areas of low rainfall, few winter freezes, and alkaline soil in Arizona, New Mexico, West Texas, San Joaquin Valley of California, and parts of Mexico and South America. The primary method of infection is through inhalation of aerosolized arthrospores, although rarely, infection from a direct cutaneous inoculation is possible. The majority of infections are asymptomatic and self-resolving. Symptomatic patients typically present as community-acquired pneumonia with symptoms of fever, rash, and flu like symptoms. Uncommonly, in about 1% of infections, hematogenous extra pulmonary systemic dissemination involving skin, musculoskeletal system, and meninges occur. Involvement of the spine can range from discitis and paravertebral soft tissue infection to vertebral body erosion and neural compression [1–3]. Extrapulmonary disseminated coccidioidomycosis with involvement of the spine, either localized or multiple segments is treated with antifungal drugs and/or surgical treatment. In this article, we present cases of spinal coccidioidomycosis treated at our institution and review the current literature.

2. Materials and Methods

We conducted a retrospective review of medical records of all patients treated for spinal coccidioidomycosis at our institution. We queried the medical records of all in-patient admissions in our institution between January 2009 and December 2018 for the diagnosis of spinal coccidioidomycosis. We retrospectively reviewed patient demographics, clinical characteristics, presenting symptoms, radiological features, management, and outcomes of all patients treated for spinal coccidioidomycoses. Radiographic features of infection in the spine including the location of infection, characteristics of magnetic resonance imaging (MRI), number of vertebral segments involved, and involvement of neural elements and paraspinal structures were studied. An Institutional Review Board was done at our institution.

3. Results

A total of 373 patients of coccidioidomycosis (pulmonary or systemic disseminated) were treated from January 2009 to December 2018 at our institution. There were three cases (male = 3, 0.80% of patients) of coccidioidomycosis infection of the spine during the same period. All three patients presented with pain symptoms in the spine, and two patients had neurological deficits. We describe the presentation, management and outcomes in these cases.

3.1. Case Illustration 1

A 28-year-old man presented with a one-month history of lower back pain, worsening shortness of breath, and intermittent fevers over a period of the month. He was initially treated with azithromycin at an outside facility, which failed to resolve his symptoms. The back pain was progressively severe and radiated to both lower extremities, limiting his ambulation. He had no history of sick contacts, travel, or history of exposure to tuberculosis patients. Initial treatment included empiric antibiotics and screening tests for HIV, tuberculosis with PCR, legionella, and a endemic mycosis serology panel that included histoplasmosis, blastomycosis, and coccidioidomycosis. A CT scan of the chest revealed lucencies throughout mid-thoracic spine with adjacent prominence of paraspinal soft tissues suggestive of osteomyelitis and discitis. MRI of the T spine revealed abnormal marrow enhancement seen with varying degrees of paraspinal soft tissue enhancement, the most significant being at T6 where diffuse marrow enhancement and vertebral height loss was seen (Figure 1a,b). A biopsy of the lesion confirmed the coccidioidomycosis (Figure 1c). He was initiated on antifungal therapy—voriconazole and amphotericin B—followed by surgical debridement and stabilization.

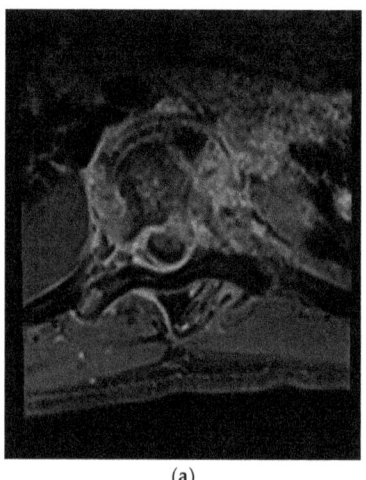

(a)

Figure 1. *Cont.*

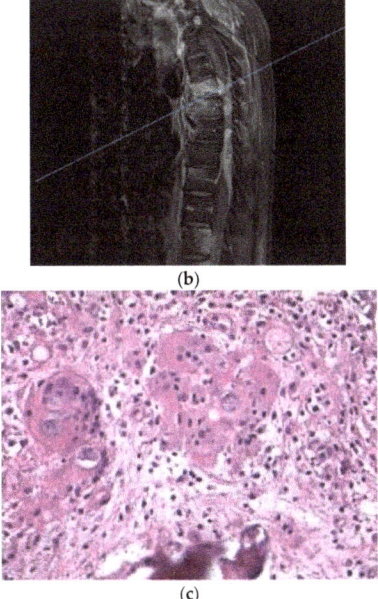

Figure 1. (**a**) Axial T1-weighted magnetic resonance (MR) images with contrast showing extensive vertebral body and soft tissue enhancement with compression of the spinal canal at T6. (**b**) Sagittal T1-weighted MR Images with contrast showing extensive enhancement throughout the vertebral bodies and soft tissue but most significantly at T6–7. (**c**) Hematoxylin and eosin (H&E) staining of the thoracic bone specimen showing acute osteomyelitis with abundant coccidioides organisms. Multinucleated giant cells with engulfed coccidioides spherules is a characteristic finding. Abundant acute inflammatory changes was noted in the marrow cavity.

He underwent bilateral T7–9 laminectomies and foraminotomies for decompression of the spinal cord. The abscess was identified and noted to be fibrous and adherent to the duramater. Caseating tissue was noted epidurally extending more in to the left lateral recess. Debridement and washout of all extraneous infected tissue was performed. Four days later, the patient underwent a transnasal approach for incision and drainage of pre-clival and retropharyngeal abscess. At 1-year follow-up, he continued to have moderate to severe axial sharp pain in the neck and lower back. An MRI demonstrated persistent marrow changes in lumbar spine and pelvis, as noted previously.

3.2. Case Illustration 2

A 62-year-old man with past medical history of pulmonary fungal infection presented with a seven-month history of back pain. He was initially diagnosed with coccidioides pneumonia seven years ago and was placed on a fluconazole long-term treatment, which was later discontinued by another physician due to renal adverse effects. He presented with symptoms of severe lower back pain, which exacerbated when sitting or lying down. The symptoms of pain were associated with weakness in the lower extremities and poor balance while walking. He had chronic non-radiating back pain. MRI of the lumbar spine revealed L1–2 discitis and osteomyelitis with a paraspinal abscess (Figure 2a). Antibiotics therapy and fluconazole were started preliminarily. An image-guided interventional biopsy demonstrated coccidioidomycosis infection. Neurologically, having motor deficits and severe pain with imaging confirming compression of neural elements warranted surgical treatment. A lateral approach to the lumbar spine was undertaken to perform corpectomy of the L1 and L2 vertebral bodies along with discectomy and insertion of an expandable cage with a morselized bone graft. This construct was reinforced with a posterior instrumented fusion extending two segments superiorly and inferiorly (Figure 2b). The intraoperative specimen showed coccidiodes spherules within the bone specimen, consistent with dissemination of the infection to the spine (Figure 2c).

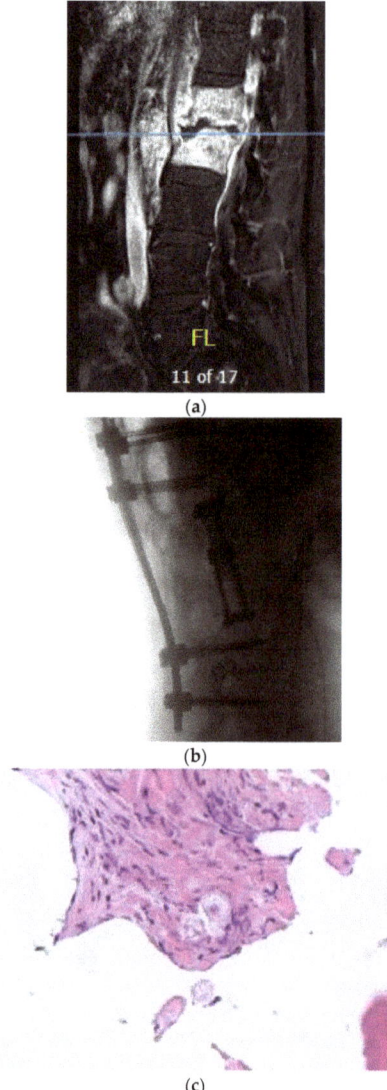

Figure 2. (**a**) Sagittal T1-weighted MR images with contrast showing extensive disc space destruction at L1–2 with epidural enhancement. (**b**) Sagittal T–L junction X-ray showing postoperative changes with a L1–2 corpectomy and instrumented fusion. (**c**) H&E staining of the intraoperative vertebral body specimen demonstrating the spherules within bone indicating osteomyelitis.

3.3. Case Illustration 3

A 54-year-old man with a past medical history of hypertension, C3–4 osteomyelitis, prevertebral/epidural abscess, and left septic knee who presented initially to his primary care physician with left upper extremity and lower extremity weakness, left knee pain, and lab results remarkable for elevated white blood cell count. Infectious disease workup and joint aspiration of the left sternoclavicular joint infection with coccidioidomycosis were confirmed. He was treated with intravenous fluconazole and vancomycin. The MRI and CT scan for evaluating the weakness revealed osteomyelitis/discitis of C3–4 and a focal epidural abscess (Figure 3a,b). In addition, he was diagnosed with a left septic knee and underwent aspiration of joint effusion. A repeat MRI of the cervical spine later revealed improvement in the size and inflammation of the epidural abscess, and the patient was discharged on IV liposomal amphotericin B 50 mg per day. A few weeks later, the patient presented to the emergency room with fever, tachycardia, and tingling in the bilateral upper extremities. MRI of the cervical spine revealed retrolisthesis of C3 and C4, spinal canal stenosis, and cord compression due to extension of the epidural abscess into the level of the C5 vertebra. Furthermore, extensive discitis and osteomyelitis with collection in both the epidural and prevertebral regions were noted. The patient was clinically noted to have motor weakness in the left upper extremity and was transferred to our institution for a higher level of care and management. The abscess was surgically treated with incision and drainage of the prevertebral abscess, a C4 corpectomy, C3–5 fusion with placement of a cage, and an anterior plate from C3–5. Figure 3a shows the Coccidiodes spherules in the ventral epidural abscess. During the hospitalization, he also underwent several debridement procedures and arthrocentesis of his infected left knee.

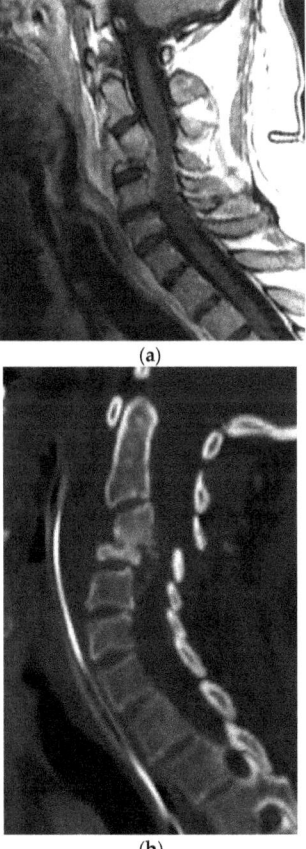

(a)

(b)

Figure 3. *Cont.*

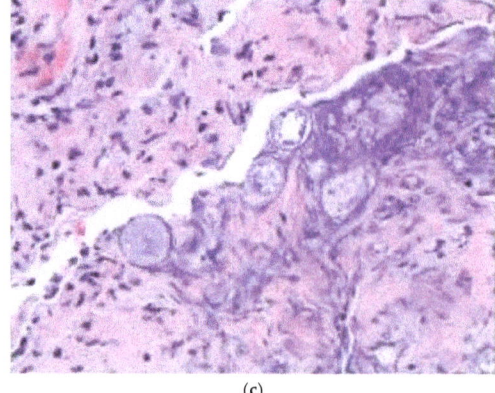

(c)

Figure 3. (a) Sagittal T1-weighted MR images with contrast showing extensive disc space destruction at C3-4 with epidural enhancement. (b) Sagittal cervical spine CT showing postoperative erosion of the C4 vertebral body significant retrolisthesis of C3 onto C4. (c) H&E stain of the cervical spinal pathologic specimen demonstrating the *Coccidioides* spherules within soft tissue, which is morphologically compatible with coccidioidomycotic osteomyelitis.

4. Discussion

Coccidioidomycosis is a fungal infection that is asymptomatic in a majority of patients. Patients with symptomatic infection generally present with isolated pulmonary involvement manifesting as a flu-like syndrome—headache, night sweats, rash, arthralgia, and myalgia. Disseminated infection via bloodstream and lymphatics is less common and is noted frequently in immunocompromised patients. Extrapulmonary disease to the musculoskeletal system has a predilection for the axial bones and commonly involves the vertebral bodies.

Musculoskeletal involvement is a feature in about half of the disseminated forms with about 2–3% of this population being symptomatic. Vertebral and neurological involvement seems to be more common among Asian and African-American populations. Spinal coccidioidomycosis should be diagnosed early to prevent the local spread of infection and involvement of neural elements. Clinically, vertebral coccidioidomycosis commonly presents with symptoms of back pain or neck pain with associated radiculopathy, sensory disturbances, and motor weakness [4]. Both symptomatic and asymptomatic pulmonary coccidioidomycosis infections can lead to spinal coccidioidomycosis, although it is more frequent in patients with symptomatic pulmonary infection [5]. Therefore, patients with symptoms of back pain and associated neurological symptoms such as motor weakness or sensory symptoms, with travel or residence history in endemic areas should be evaluated for coccidioidomycosis [1,6,7]. *Coccidioides* species titer serological tests must be obtained early and is helpful in establishing the diagnosis. IgM elevation is noted in 1–3 weeks of infection, and IgG elevation occurs in 2–28 weeks, with titers greater than 1 in 128 is suggestive of bone or joint involvement [3,5]. Erythrocyte sedimentation rates and C-reactive protein, though not sensitive or specific to coccidioidomycosis, are frequently elevated.

MRI, though not diagnostic, can demonstrate erosive defects in vertebrae and endplates and vertebral body collapse or paraspinal extension in more advanced cases. An MRI is more sensitive than a CT scan or plain radiographic films at detecting early changes due to infection. Typically, both active and necrotic lesions display T1 lengthening with contrast enhancement. Active lesions are hyper-intense in T2-weighted sequences. MRI cannot differentiate the findings in coccidioidomycosis, vertebral metastasis, tuberculosis, and other infectious diseases. Biopsy of vertebral lesions, generally CT-guided, to detect *Coccidioides immitis/posadasii* spherules is required for definitive diagnosis even with known involvement of other organ systems to rule out other alternative causes for spinal involvement.

Several stains, including hematoxylin and eosin and periodic acid-Schiff stains (PAS), calcofluor white fluorescent, and Gomori methenamine silver, can identify the pathogen microscopically [1,6].

4.1. Medical Therapy

Spinal coccidioidomycosis is managed with pharmacologic and surgical treatment. All symptomatic patients with spinal involvement are initiated on antifungal therapy for a period of 12 to 18 months [1,2,8–10]. Untreated patients can progress to sepsis and eventual death, and therefore all patients require medical therapy.

Amphotericin has been used conventionally to treat coccidioidomycosis. Antimycotic treatment with azoles is more commonly being used as first line therapy to avoid the adverse effects of amphotericin, especially in cases with localized spinal infections. Fluconazole is most commonly used azole antifungal treatment for coccidioidomycosis. Other azole treatments include voriconazole and itraconazole. Voriconazole has shown to be effective in treating disseminated infection in contrast to fluconazole or itraconazole [5]. More recently, posaconazole has demonstrated efficacy with superior osseous penetration [11,12]. Immunocompromised patients and patients with meningitis are treated lifelong with azoles [1,7,10]. Patients who respond poorly to azoles will them typically progress to polytherapy that includes amphotericin in addition to multiple azoles. Compliance with multiple medical therapy is a challenge in treating these patients, which is a major cause of relapse of infection, although progressive infection and decline are not uncommon while adhering to therapy [5,13–20].

4.2. Surgical Treatment

Surgical treatment is indicated in patients with severe disease or who are poor respondents to medical therapy or have intractable pain, the presence of neurological deficits, compression, or structural spinal instability [1,5,9,21–23]. Surgical treatment with medical therapy is noted to be effective in alleviating pain and symptoms and limiting the disease compared to medical therapy alone [2,5,9,24,25]. Titanium hardware has been safely used for spinal stabilization in coccidioidomycosis as with other spinal infections. These have been demonstrated to be resistant to biofilm formation and aid in eradication of infection by limiting spinal mobility in the involved segments [1,26–31]. We have summarized the treatment details and relevant outcomes in some of the larger case series (with greater than 10 patients) reported in the literature (Table 1).

Interval MRI should be used to assess for patients' response to therapy. Surgical treatment is indicated in patients with spinal instability, neurological deficits or motor weakness, abscess formation, or osteolysis. Poor response to antifungal therapy or continued intractable pain with an attributable focus of infection are also additional indications for surgery. Surgical treatment involves debridement of infected tissue and instrumented fusion.

Table 1. Summary of case reports of coccidioidomycotic osteomyelitis.

Study	No. of Patients	Medical Treatment Used	Surgical and Medical Treatment (No. of Patients)	Mean Age/Range (year)	Outcomes
Winter et al., (1978) [18]	12	IV amphotericin	Surgical + medical	2–35	Two patients died—one died five years later of coccidioidal meningitis, one died of fulminant spinal infection. One patient had paraplegia from thoracic spondylitis.
Zeppa et al., (1996) [20]	10	High dose IV liposomal amphotericin B. IV antibiotics with vancomycin and Zosyn for presumed bacterial infection	Surgical + medical (1)	33	Successfully treated then developed recurrence two years later despite being on suppressive oral antifungal treatment.
Herron et al., (1997) [25]	16	IV amphotericin B	Medical only group, medical + surgical group	40	Nine patients who had surgical and medical treatment had remission. Others were in medical only who had lost to follow-up.
Wrobel et al., (2001) [19]	23	Amphotericin and/or fluconazole	Surgical and medical	9–62	One: worsened postoperatively. One: reoperation needed. Four: died, 2/2 to fungemia. Most of the 15 surviving patients needed long-term antifungal treatment for extraspinal and spinal foci.
Kakarla et al., (2011) [9]	27	Amphotericin B, fluconazole, or voriconazole	Medical and surgical treatment	41.4	Follow-up for 19/27 patients: 16 improved 1 stable 1 worsened 1 died
Szeyko et al., (2012) [5]	39	All patients received triazole and 20 also received amphotericin B (usually early in the course)	Medical and surgical	35	None of the patients developed recurrence or refractory infection at the site of debridement. Six patients relapsed after stopping antifungal treatment.

5. Conclusions

Disseminated coccidioidomycosis can lead to spondylitis that can present as discitis or localized spinal or paraspinal abscesses. Early diagnosis with serologic tests helps in preventing disease extension and systemic complications. Medical management with antifungal therapy is the first line of treatment for disseminated spinal coccidioidomycosis. In cases of spinal involvement leading to mechanical instability, compression of neural elements, and intractable pain, surgical treatment with debridement and/or instrumented stabilization is indicated.

Author Contributions: conceptualization, E.K. and D.R.; methodology, E.K.; software, E.K.; validation, E.K., D.R., and N.S.; formal analysis, E.K. and D.R.; investigation, E.K., D.R., and N.S.; resources, E.K. and N.S.; data curation, E.K., D.R., and N.S.; writing—original draft preparation, D.R. and E.K.; writing—review and editing, E.K.; visualization, D.R.; supervision, E.K.; project administration, E.K.

Funding: This research received no external funding.

Conflicts of Interest: The authors declare no conflict of interest.

References

1. El Abd, O.H.; Fusco, H.N.; Gomba, L.; Lew, M.; Jenis, L. Coccidioidomycosis infection presenting with thoracic spinal pain. *PM R.* **2012**, *4*, 450–455. [CrossRef] [PubMed]
2. Reach, P.; Paugam, A.; Kahan, A.; Allanore, Y.; Wipff, J. Coccidioidomycosis of the spine in an immunocompetent patient. *Jt. Bone Spine* **2010**, *77*, 611–613. [CrossRef] [PubMed]
3. Saubolle, M.A.; McKellar, P.P.; Sussland, D. Epidemiologic, clinical, and diagnostic aspects of coccidioidomycosis. *J. Clin. Microbiol.* **2007**, *45*, 26–30. [CrossRef] [PubMed]
4. Baaj, A.A.; Martirosyan, N.L.; Skoch, J.M.; Zaninovich, O.; Zoccali, C.; Galgiani, J.N. A paradigm for the evaluation and management of spinal coccidioidomycosis. *Surg. Neurol. Int.* **2015**, *6*, 107. [CrossRef] [PubMed]
5. Szeyko, L.A.; Taljanovic, M.S.; Dzioba, R.B.; Rapiejko, J.L.; Adam, R.D. Vertebral Coccidioidomycosis: Presentation and Multidisciplinary Management. *Am. J. Med.* **2012**, *125*, 304–314. [CrossRef] [PubMed]
6. Saubolle, M.A. Laboratory Aspects in the Diagnosis of Coccidioidomycosis. *Ann. New York Acad. Sci.* **2007**, *1111*, 301–314. [CrossRef] [PubMed]
7. Tan, L.A.; Kasliwal, M.K.; Nag, S.; O'Toole, J.E.; Traynelis, V.C. Rapidly progressive quadriparesis heralding disseminated coccidioidomycosis in an immunocompetent patient. *J. Clin. Neurosci.* **2014**, *21*, 1049–1051. [CrossRef]
8. Jackson, F.E.; Kent, D.; Clare, F. Quadriplegia Caused by Involvement of Cervical Spine with Coccidioides immitis. *J. Neurosurg.* **1964**, *21*, 512–515. [CrossRef]
9. Kakarla, U.K.; Kalani, M.Y.; Sharma, G.K.; Sonntag, V.K.; Theodore, N. Surgical management of coccidioidomycosis of the spine: Clinical article. *J. Neurosurgery Spine* **2011**, *15*, 441–446. [CrossRef]
10. Limper, A.H.; Knox, K.S.; Sarosi, G.A.; Ampel, N.M.; Bennett, J.E.; Catanzaro, A.; Davies, S.F.; Dismukes, W.E.; Hage, C.A.; Marr, K.A.; et al. An Official American Thoracic Society Statement: Treatment of Fungal Infections in Adult Pulmonary and Critical Care Patients. *Am. J. Respir. Crit. Care Med.* **2011**, *183*, 96–128. [CrossRef]
11. Anstead, G.M.; Corcoran, G.; Lewis, J.; Berg, D.; Graybill, J.R. Refractory Coccidioidomycosis Treated with Posaconazole. *Clin. Infect. Dis.* **2005**, *40*, 1770–1776. [CrossRef] [PubMed]
12. Catanzaro, A.; Cloud, G.A.; Stevens, D.A.; Levine, B.E.; Williams, P.L.; Johnson, R.H.; Rendon, A.; Mirels, L.F.; Lutz, J.E.; Holloway, M.; et al. Safety, Tolerance, and Efficacy of Posaconazole Therapy in Patients with Nonmeningeal Disseminated or Chronic Pulmonary Coccidioidomycosis. *Clin. Infect. Dis.* **2007**, *45*, 562–568. [CrossRef] [PubMed]
13. Bried, J.M.; Galgiani, J.N. Coccidioides immitis infections in bones and joints. *Clin. Orthop. Relat. Res.* **1986**, *211*, 235–243. [CrossRef]
14. Centers for Disease Control and Prevention (CDC). Increase in reported coccidioidomycosis—United States, 1998–2011. *MMWR Morb. Mortal. Wkly. Rep.* **2013**, *62*, 217–221.
15. Copeland, B.; White, D.; Buenting, J. Coccidioidomycosis of the Head and Neck. *Ann. Otol. Rhinol. Laryngol.* **2003**, *112*, 98–101. [CrossRef] [PubMed]

16. Lewicky, Y.M.; Roberto, R.F.; Curtin, S.L. The unique complications of coccidioidomycosis of the spine: A detailed time line of disease progression and suppression. *Spine* **2004**, *29*, 435–441. [CrossRef]
17. McGahan, J.P.; Graves, D.S.; Palmer, P.E. Coccidioidal spondylitis: Usual and unusual radiographic manifestations. *Radiology* **1980**, *136*, 5–9. [CrossRef] [PubMed]
18. Winter, W.G., Jr.; Larson, R.K.; Zettas, J.P.; Libke, R. Coccidioidal spondylitis. *J. Bone Joint Surgery Am. Vol.* **1978**, *60*, 240–244. [CrossRef]
19. Wrobel, C.J.; Chappell, E.T.; Taylor, W. Clinical presentation, radiological findings, and treatment results of coccidioidomycosis involving the spine: Report on 23 cases. *J. Neurosurgery Spine* **2001**, *95*, 33–39. [CrossRef]
20. Zeppa, M.A.; Laorr, A.; Greenspan, A.; McGahan, J.P.; Steinbach, L.S. Skeletal coccidioidomycosis: Imaging findings in 19 patients. *Skelet. Radiol.* **1996**, *25*, 337–343. [CrossRef]
21. Halpern, E.M.; Bacon, S.A.; Kitagawa, T.; Lewis, S.J. Posterior Transdiscal Three-Column Shortening in the Surgical Treatment of Vertebral Discitis/Osteomyelitis With Collapse. *Spine* **2010**, *35*, 1316–1322. [CrossRef] [PubMed]
22. Lange, T.; Schulte, T.L.; Bullmann, V. Two recurrences of adjacent spondylodiscitis after initial surgical intervention with posterior stabilization, debridement, and reconstruction of the anterior column in a patient with spondylodiscitis: A case report. *Spine* **2010**, *35*, 804–810. [CrossRef] [PubMed]
23. Lee, D.-G.; Park, K.B.; Kang, D.-H.; Hwang, S.H.; Jung, J.M.; Han, J.W. A Clinical Analysis of Surgical Treatment for Spontaneous Spinal Infection. *J. Korean Neurosurg. Soc.* **2007**, *42*, 317–325. [CrossRef] [PubMed]
24. Bisla, R.S.; Taber, T.H., Jr. Coccidioidomycosis of bone and joints. *Clin. Orthop. Relat. Res.* **1976**, *121*, 196–204. [CrossRef]
25. Herron, L.D.; Kissel, P.; Smilovitz, D. Treatment of coccidioidal spinal infection: Experience in 16 cases. *J. Spinal Disord.* **1997**, *10*, 215–222. [CrossRef] [PubMed]
26. Akers, K.S.; The Infectious Disease Clinical Research Program Trauma Infectious Disease Outcomes Study Group; Mende, K.; A Cheatle, K.; Zera, W.C.; Yu, X.; Beckius, M.L.; Aggarwal, D.; Li, P.; Sanchez, C.J.; et al. Biofilms and persistent wound infections in United States military trauma patients: A case–control analysis. *BMC Infect. Dis.* **2014**, *14*, 190. [CrossRef] [PubMed]
27. Sheehan, E.; McKenna, J.; Mulhall, K.J.; Marks, P.; McCormack, D. Adhesion of Staphylococcus to orthopaedic metals, an in vivo study. *J. Orthop. Res.* **2004**, *22*, 39–43. [CrossRef]
28. Kostakioti, M.; Hadjifrangiskou, M.; Hultgren, S.J. Bacterial Biofilms: Development, Dispersal, and Therapeutic Strategies in the Dawn of the Postantibiotic Era. *Cold Spring Harb. Perspect. Med.* **2013**, *3*, a010306. [CrossRef]
29. Liljenqvist, U.; Lerner, T.; Bullmann, V.; Hackenberg, L.; Halm, H.; Winkelmann, W. Titanium cages in the surgical treatment of severe vertebral osteomyelitis. *Eur. Spine J.* **2003**, *12*, 606–612. [CrossRef]
30. Sanchez, C.J.; Mende, K.; Beckius, M.L.; Akers, K.S.; Romano, D.R.; Wenke, J.C.; Murray, C.K. Biofilm formation by clinical isolates and the implications in chronic infections. *BMC Infect. Dis.* **2013**, *13*, 47. [CrossRef]
31. Trampuz, A.; Piper, K.E.; Jacobson, M.J.; Hanssen, A.D.; Unni, K.K.; Osmon, D.R.; Mandrekar, J.N.; Cockerill, F.R.; Steckelberg, J.M.; Greenleaf, J.F.; et al. Sonication of Removed Hip and Knee Prostheses for Diagnosis of Infection. *New Engl. J. Med.* **2007**, *357*, 654–663. [CrossRef] [PubMed]

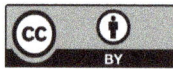

© 2019 by the authors. Licensee MDPI, Basel, Switzerland. This article is an open access article distributed under the terms and conditions of the Creative Commons Attribution (CC BY) license (http://creativecommons.org/licenses/by/4.0/).

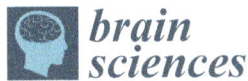

Case Report

Self Manipulated Cervical Spine Leads to Posterior Disc Herniation and Spinal Stenosis

Wyatt McGilvery [1,*], Marc Eastin [2], Anish Sen [2] and Maciej Witkos [1]

1. Department of Emergency Medicine, Loma Linda University Medical Center, Loma Lind, CA 92354, USA; mwitkos@llu.edu
2. Department of Neurosurgery, Loma Linda University Medical Center, Loma Lind, CA 92354, USA; meastin@llu.edu (M.E.); asen@llu.edu (A.S.)
* Correspondence: wyattmcgilvery@gmail.com

Received: 29 April 2019; Accepted: 27 May 2019; Published: 29 May 2019

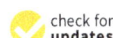

Abstract: The authors report a case in which a 38-year-old male who presented himself to the emergency department with a chief complaint of cervical neck pain and paresthesia radiating from the right pectoral region down his distal right arm following self-manipulation of the patient's own cervical vertebrae. Initial emergency department imaging via cervical x-ray and magnetic resonance imaging (MRI) without contrast revealed no cervical fractures; however, there was evidence of an acute cervical disc herniation (C3–C7) with severe herniation and spinal stenosis located at C5–C6. Immediate discectomy at C5–C6 and anterior arthrodesis was conducted in order to decompress the cervical spinal cord. Acute traumatic cervical disc herniation is rare in comparison to disc herniation due to the chronic degradation of the posterior annulus fibrosus and nucleus pulposus. Traumatic cervical hernias usually arise due to a very large external force causing hyperflexion or hyperextension of the cervical vertebrae. However, there have been reports of cervical injury arising from cervical spinal manipulation therapy (SMT) where a licensed professional applies a rotary force component. This can be concerning, considering that 12 million Americans receive SMT annually (Powell, F.C.; Hanigan, W.C.; Olivero, W.C. A risk/benefit analysis of spinal manipulation therapy for relief of lumbar or cervical pain. *Neurosurgery* **1993**, *33*, 73–79.). This case study involved an individual who was able to apply enough rotary force to his own cervical vertebrae, causing severe neurological damage requiring surgical intervention. Individuals with neck pain should be advised of the complications of SMT, and provided with alternative treatment methods, especially if one is willing to self manipulate.

Keywords: cervical disk herniation; spinal stenosis; neurosurgery; discectomy; arthrodesis; anterior approach; self manipulation; cervical spine; spinal manipulation therapy; acute trauma

1. Introduction

The etiology of cervical herniated nucleus pulposus, or herniated discs, most often arise due to age related degenerative properties such as dehydration and weakening of the posterior annulus fibrosus and nucleus pulposus, ultimately leading to posterior disc herniation and protrusion into the spinal canal. A lesser common etiology of cervical herniated nucleus is traumatic, usually associated with a high energy external force resulting in extreme hyperflexion or hyperextension of the cervical vertebrae [1]. However, we are currently unaware of any other case where self manipulation (forced external rotation) of one's own cervical vertebrae has led to traumatic posterior cervical disc protrusion and severe central spinal stenosis requiring immediate surgical intervention. This case study has been submitted to, and approved by Loma Linda University Health's Institutional Review Board (IRB) in order to ensure all ethical criterion has been met.

2. Case Report

A 38-year-old male with a remote history penetrating neck trauma in 2013 presented himself to the emergency department with a chief complaint of acute posterior cervical neck pain and paresthesia. Prior to the onset of acute neck pain, the patient had attempted to manipulate his own cervical vertebrae in order to relieve himself of a continuously nagging "crick in the neck." After his first attempt of using both hands (one hand on the anterolateral aspect of his mandible, and the other hand on his occipital region) to apply external rotation and torsion of his cervical vertebrae, he heard a loud crunching sound, followed by immediate neck pain. This neck pain worsened with movement, associated with unilateral radiating pain and paresthesia down his right arm and extending to his right pectoral region, whole body numbness below his shoulders, and a throbbing component of pain when at rest. Patient denied any other neurological symptoms including headache, nausea, vomiting, blurry vision, changes in hearing, loss of balance, aphasia, loss of extremity strength, fecal or urinary incontinence or retention, and denies any use of aspirin or any other anticoagulation medications.

Physical examination found that the patient had 5/5 strength throughout except a 4+/5 distal right hand strength. The patient also had decreased sensation to light touch below the neck, which was worse on the right side. The patient did not have clonus or Hoffman's sign, no Babinski's sign, nor hyperreflexia. Initial MRI results showed a large 5–6 mm traumatic right paracentral posterior disc protrusion with disruption of the posterior disc annulus at the C5–C6 level with associated severe central spinal stenosis and ligamentous damage to the posterior longitudinal ligament (PLL). There was also mild to moderate central spinal stenosis secondary to smaller disc protrusions at the C3–C4 and C6–C7 levels (Figure 1). Initial MRI showed no osseous fractures of the vertebrae, nor asymmetry in the alignment of any faucet joints.

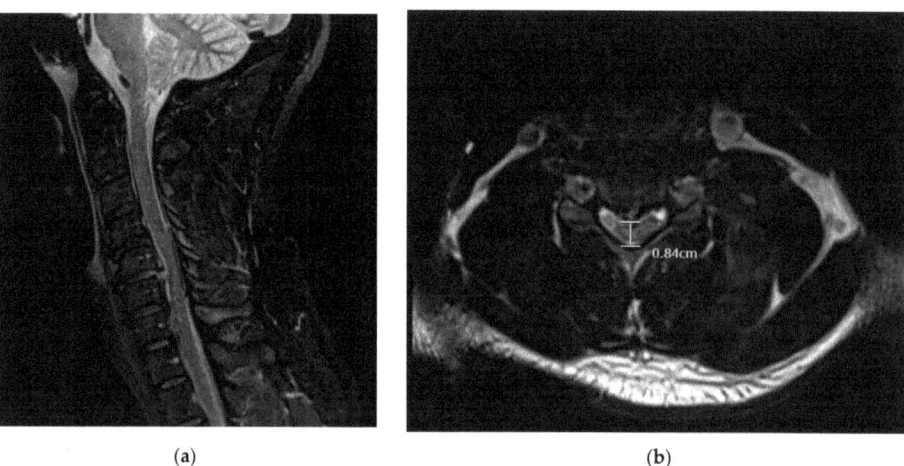

(a)   (b)

Figure 1. Preoperative MRI (STIR sequence sagittal (Figure 1a) and T2 axial (Figure 1b)) taken in the emergency department shows the pathology of C5–C6 posterior acute cervical disc herniation with increased signal in the posterior longitudinal ligament and severe spinal cord compression with cord signal change status post self-manipulation of neck. The encircled area also shows the protrusion of the posterior herniated disc causing spinal stenosis. MRI = magnetic resonance imaging.

A discectomy and arthrodesis surgical intervention was opted to be performed on the patient due to myelopathy upon examination. In addition to this, the patient had radiculopathy and ligamentous injury.

3. Surgical Interventions

Given the patient's presenting symptoms and neurological deficits (hand weakness, numbness), combined with the MRI findings of an acute disc herniation with severe spinal cord compression, neurosurgery was consulted. As the patient had acute neurological changes, it was recommended that the patient undergo urgent surgery for an anterior C5–C6 discectomy and arthrodesis.

After the patient was placed under general anesthesia, electrodes were placed for motor-evoked potential and somatosensory-evoked potentials. Baseline potentials were then obtained and remained stable throughout the entire procedure. A transverse right anterior neck incision was made at the C5–C6 level, confirmed by intraoperative X-ray. Once appropriate anatomical structures were divided and retracted, a large disc fragment was encountered between C5–C6 and removed below the PLL. Decompression was then confirmed with a nerve hook. A 6 mm cadaveric structural allograft was then sized and positioned with X-ray. Meticulous disc space hemostasis was obtained.

Copious irrigation was then performed prior to a 12 mm anterior cervical plate being secured with 4.0 ×16 mm screws in C5 and variable screws in C6.

The patient tolerated the procedure well and intraoperative X-rays confirmed proper placement of the plate screws and interbody device. The incision was then irrigated with antibiotic irrigation and closed in a layered fashion. The patient was then extubated and transported to postoperative recovery in a stable condition.

A postoperative CT scan confirmed the proper anterior fixation of the plate screws, interbody device, and bone graft placement following the patient's discectomy and arthrodesis (Figure 2). Postoperative anterior and lateral X-rays (Figure 3b,a respectively) were also obtained in order to visualize and confirm proper placement of the anterior cervical plate and evaluation of alignment.

On follow up at one month, the patient had resolution of his numbness and paresthesia, however, he continued to note posterior midline neck pain. He reported cannabinoid and methamphetamine use despite discussion to avoid drugs while fusion was occurring. He was subsequently lost to follow up.

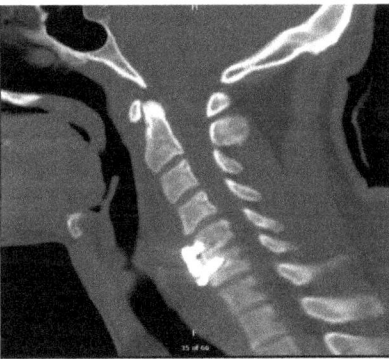

Figure 2. Postoperative CT scan showing spinal cord decompression following surgical discectomy and anterior arthrodesis of the C5–C6 vertebrae. CT scan = computerized tomography scan.

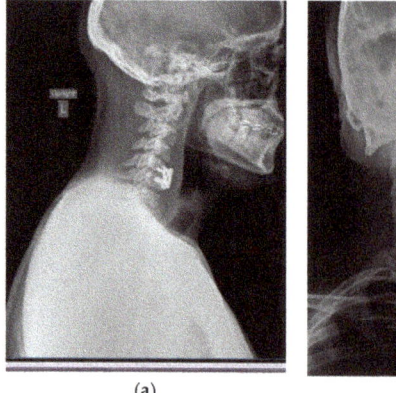

Figure 3. Postoperative X-ray showing postsurgical changes related to anterior fusion at C5–C6, with interval decrease in prevertebral soft tissue swelling. C1–C7 are visualized on the lateral view (Figure 3a) for evaluation of alignment. There is straightening of the normal cervical lordosis. Alignment is otherwise grossly unremarkable when allowing for patient rotation. Anterior instrumentation is noted at C5–C6 on both lateral and anterior (Figure 3b) views.

4. Discussion

When researching other published literature for similar cases regarding cervical manipulation resulting in cervical disc herniation and subsequent spinal stenosis, few reports were found. However, publications like that by Yang [2] indicate the possibilities of cervical spinal stenosis that can arise from cervical SMT. The most common injuries associated with cervical SMT all seem to be reported occurring at the C5–C6 level.

It is our belief that patients should be advised of alternative therapy methods such as physiotherapy when discussing the treatment of acute cervical neck pain due to the unusually high risk/benefit ratio of cervical SMT[4].

Our case study is relatively unique, as there have been no other reports to our knowledge of the self-manipulation of one's own cervical spine leading to severe acute disc herniation and neurological deficits. Most reports of this sort of injury have been attested due to age related degenerative factors, and a few cervical SMTs provided by other licensed professionals. In addition to this, it is known that 85% of all patients suffering from symptoms of an acute herniated disc will resolve themselves within 8–12 days without the need of specific treatment [3]. The fact that our patient's pathology included a severe herniation causing spinal stenosis with neurological deficits in need of urgent neurosurgical intervention further attests to the uniqueness of this case.

5. Conclusions

Self manipulation of the cervical vertebrae may result in acute traumatic cervical disc herniation, severe enough to result in focal neurological deficits. Individuals who feel the need to stretch their neck in an external torsion or rotary manner should be educated in the possible dangers of doing so. Individuals presenting with acute neck or arm pain, leg pain, paresthesia, or other neurological symptomatology post self cervical manipulation or "stretching" should be evaluated for possible cervical disc protrusions and spinal stenosis via MRI.

Author Contributions: W.M. is noted as the primary author and contributor responsible for external research/literature review and constructing the manuscript. Both M.E. and A.S. were the consulting neurosurgeons, and responsible for the surgical interventions and explanations. M.W. was the overseeing physician/author responsible for the complete paper oversight, management, and for obtaining ethical consent through Loma Linda University Medical Center IRB.

Funding: This research received no external funding.

Conflicts of Interest: The authors declare no conflict of interest.

References

1. Suetsuna, F.; Okudera, Y.; Tanaka, T.; Tamura, T. Spinal cord injury due to cervical disc herniation caused by bench pressing. *J. Spine* **2014**, *3*, 154. [CrossRef]
2. Yang, H.S.; Oh, Y.M.; Eun, J.P. Cervical intradural disc herniation causing progressive quadriparesis after spinal manipulation therapy: A case report and literature review. *Medicine (Baltimore)* **2016**, *95*, 2797. [CrossRef] [PubMed]
3. Dulebohn, S.C.; Massa, R.N.; Mesfin, F.B. Disc Herniation. Available online: https://www.ncbi.nlm.nih.gov/books/NBK441822/ (accessed on 15 February 2019).

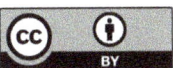

© 2019 by the authors. Licensee MDPI, Basel, Switzerland. This article is an open access article distributed under the terms and conditions of the Creative Commons Attribution (CC BY) license (http://creativecommons.org/licenses/by/4.0/).

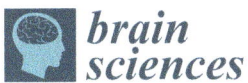

Case Report

Benign Giant Cell Lesion of C1 Lateral Mass: A Case Report and Literature Review

Christopher Heinrich [1], Vadim Gospodarev [2,*], Albert Kheradpour [3], Craig Zuppan [4], Clifford C. Douglas [5] and Tanya Minasian [5]

1. Loma Linda University School of Medicine, Loma Linda, CA 92354, USA; ckheinrich@llu.edu
2. Center for Perinatal Biology, Department of Basic Sciences, Loma Linda University, 11234 Anderson Street, Room 2567, Loma Linda, CA 92354, USA
3. Department of Pediatric Hematology/Oncology, Loma Linda University Medical Center, 11234 Anderson Street, Loma Linda, CA 92354, USA; AKheradp@llu.edu
4. Department of Pathology, Loma Linda University Medical Center, 11234 Anderson Street, Loma Linda, CA 92354, USA; CZuppan@llu.edu
5. Department of Neurosurgery, Loma Linda University Medical Center, 11234 Anderson Street, Room 2556, Loma Linda, CA 92354, USA; CCDougla@llu.edu (C.C.D.); TMinasian@llu.edu (T.M.)
* Correspondence: vgospodarev@llu.edu; Tel.: +1-909-558-4419

Received: 24 March 2019; Accepted: 7 May 2019; Published: 8 May 2019

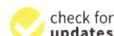

Abstract: Primary osseous tumors of the spinal column account for approximately 1% of the total number of spinal tumors found in the pediatric patient population. The authors present a case of a C1 benign giant cell lesion that was incidentally found in a 15-year-old patient. A transoral biopsy was performed followed by treatment with denosumab, with definitive management in the form of transoral tumor resection with subsequent occiput-cervical three posterior instrumented fusion. The patient tolerated all of the procedures well, as there were no post-operative complications, discharged home neurologically intact and was eager to return to school when assessed during a follow-up visit in clinic. Osteolytic lesions affecting the cervical spine are rare in the pediatric population. It is of utmost importance to have sufficient background knowledge in order to formulate a differential diagnosis, as well as an understanding of principles underlying surgical techniques required to prevent occipital-cervical instability in this patient population. The information presented will guide surgical decision-making by identifying the patient population that would benefit from neurosurgical interventions to stabilize the atlantoaxial junction, in the context of rare osteolytic conditions affecting the cervical spine.

Keywords: pain; spine; spinal disease; transoral; atlantoaxial; surgery

1. Introduction

Spinal tumors comprise approximately 5–10% of all pediatric central nervous system (CNS) tumors [1–3]. Primary osseous tumors of the spinal column only account for approximately 1% of the total number of spinal tumors [4]. The authors present a case of a C1 benign giant cell lesion, that was incidentally found in a 15-year-old patient. Despite the benign pathologic diagnosis, the unusual location and behavior of the lesion warranted an interesting surgical approach. Including a transoral biopsy first, followed by treatment with Denosumab, and finally definitive management in the form of transoral tumor resection with subsequent occiput-cervical three posterior instrumented fusion. Due to the complex anatomy of the atlantooccipital and atlantoaxial joint spaces and related structures, treatment of a mass in this region, whether benign or malignant, would necessitate non-surgical management as first-line treatment. However, if a mass is deemed to be locally destructive, resistant to medical management, or both, then a definitive surgical approach is necessary. Regardless of treatment paradigm, effective dissolution of a lytic lesion in this region can destabilize the atlantooccipital and atlantoaxial joints endangering key neurovascular structures. Because of this, stabilization of these joints using instrumented fusion is key to prevention of patient morbidity and potential mortality.

2. Case Description

A 15-year-old female with no significant past medical history presented after being struck in the face by a ball while playing water polo. The patient felt pain in her jaw, which was the chief complaint when she presented to the emergency department. Upon neurological assessment, the patient complained of midline tenderness from the skull base to midline cervical spine over C3; denied headaches, changes in vision, speech or swallowing, extremity weakness or paresthesias. A maxillofacial computed tomography (CT) scan did not show evidence of an acute facial fracture. However, the CT scan did reveal a radiolucent, ovoid-shaped lytic lesion arising in the left lateral mass of C1, between the anterior tubercle and the transverse process. Magnetic resonance imaging (MRI) studies further confirmed an enhancing osseous lesion at the left lateral mass of C1, with cortical breach and extension into the left lateral atlantodental joint space (Figure 1). Of note, three years prior, patient had a CT cervical spine which, upon retrospective review, demonstrated a similar but much smaller lesion.

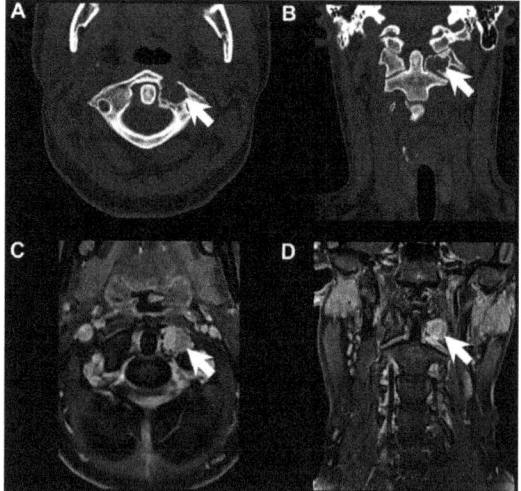

Figure 1. Pre-Operative Imaging Studies. CT of cervical spine, axial view, demonstrating the radiolucent, ovoid-shaped, lytic lesion (white arrow) arising in the left lateral mass of C1 between the anterior tubercle and the transverse process (**A**). CT of cervical spine, coronal view, demonstrating the lesion (white arrow) (**B**). Post-contrast MRI T1, axial view, demonstrating an enhancing osseous lesion (white arrow) at the left lateral mass of C1 with cortical breach and extension into the left lateral atlantodental joint space (**C**). Post-contrast MRI T1, coronal view, of the lesion (white arrow) (**D**).

Differential diagnoses underlying this vertebral cortical erosion included those of infectious etiology, as well as oncologic lesions, such as giant cell tumor of bone, aneurysmal bone cyst, osteoblastoma, osteosarcoma or even Langerhans histiocytosis (LCH). Oncology recommended that the cervical spine lesion be biopsied for tissue diagnosis. Due to the unusual location of the lesion and risk of locally aggressive pathology, or possible tumor seeding along the biopsy track, interventional radiology was unable to perform a CT guided needle biopsy. It was therefore decided that the patient would require open neurosurgical biopsy for diagnosis.

Due to the anterior and lateral location of the vertebral lesion, an anterior transoral approach to the C1 lesion was performed, in order to obtain a sufficient amount of the contrast enhancing component of the mass for pathologic diagnosis. The transoral approach was performed in a multidisciplinary fashion, during which the otolaryngology team used direct visualization, as well as stereotactic navigation, to expose the C1 anterior tubercle on the left side. Once exposure was completed, neurosurgery team utilized a matchstick burr to then drill the anterior outer cortex of C1. Multiple specimens from the fibrous tumor were taken, with curettes and pituitary forceps.

The sampled tissue did not show features of osteoblastoma or osteosarcoma, nor were there features of LCH or signs of infection. In the sampled region, the lesion consisted of a proliferation of nondescript stromal cells with intermixed multinucleated giant cells, and occasional clusters of foamy histiocytes (Figure 2). Special testing for giant cell tumor of bone (G34W staining) was negative, as was fluorescence in situ hybridization (FISH) testing for Ubiquitin Specific Peptidase 6 (USP6), making a primary form of aneurysmal bone cyst unlikely. However, due to the aggressive nature of the patient's osteolytic lesion and the significant risk for atlantoaxial instability associated with its location, it was decided to start the patient on Denosumab. Denosumab is an osteoclast inhibiting pharmaceutical agent, which was administered to the patient in order to stabilize and consolidate the lesion. Samples of the patient's lesion were also sent out to a nationally recognized expert bone pathologist, whose findings were most consistent with benign giant cell rich lesion with histiocytes.

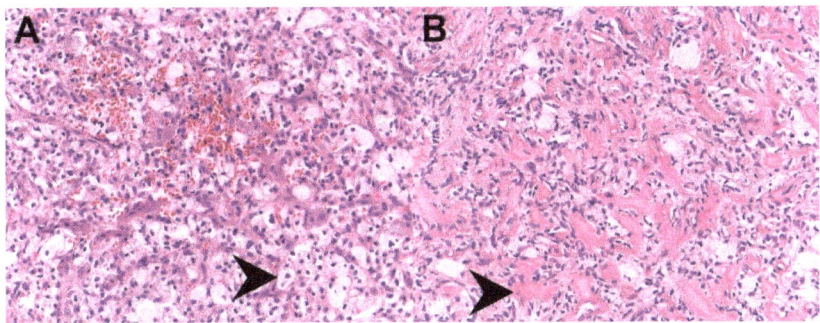

Figure 2. Histopathology. Hematoxylin and eosin (H&E) stained tissue from the initial biopsy which showed moderate prominence of histiocytic foam cells (black arrowhead), intermixed spindle cells, and scattered giant cells (**A**). H&E stained tissue following Denosumab therapy, showing disappearance of the giant cells, few foamy histiocytes, and predominance of short spindled cells in a collagenous stroma (black arrowhead) (**B**).

The patient was re-assessed three months postoperatively and MRI studies revealed that there was no interval decrease in the size of the tumor. In fact, there was a slight progression of the lesion anteriorly, despite treatment with Denosumab. After presenting the patient's case at our institution's multidisciplinary tumor board, it was decided to offer the patient a gross total resection of the offending lesion. This would inherently lead to significant atlantoaxial instability, therefore a posterior occiput to cervical three instrumented fusion was also warranted.

The transoral approach was performed in a multidisciplinary fashion, during which the otolaryngology team used direct visualization as well as stereotactic navigation, to expose the cervical vertebrae through the posterior pharynx. Fibrous tumor was identified and dissected until superior, inferior, and lateral margins of tumor resection were confirmed grossly, with fluoroscopy, and neuronavigation. Additional C1 anterior tubercle eccentric towards the right side was also taken, to include a normal bony margin. A small rim of tumor adherent to the vertebral artery was left behind. After the otolaryngology team closed the posterior pharynx, the patient was carefully turned prone, maintaining spinal precautions. Base of the occiput to cervical three was then exposed. C2 pedicle screws were placed. C3 lateral mass screws were placed. An occipital plate was sized. Screws into the occiput were placed. Fluoroscopy confirmed excellent position and spinal alignment. There were no post-operative complications and the patient was discharged home in good condition. Pathologic examination of the resected material at this time showed complete disappearance of the giant cells, due to Denosumab therapy, with the remaining lesional tissue resembling benign fibrous histiocytoma (Figure 2). Post-operative imaging studies revealed a stable posterior cervical spine construct, along with minimal rim-enhancement along the vertebral artery, as expected (Figure 3). At a three-week follow up visit in clinic, the patient's incisions were healing well, she was neurologically intact, tolerating regular diet, and was eager to return to school.

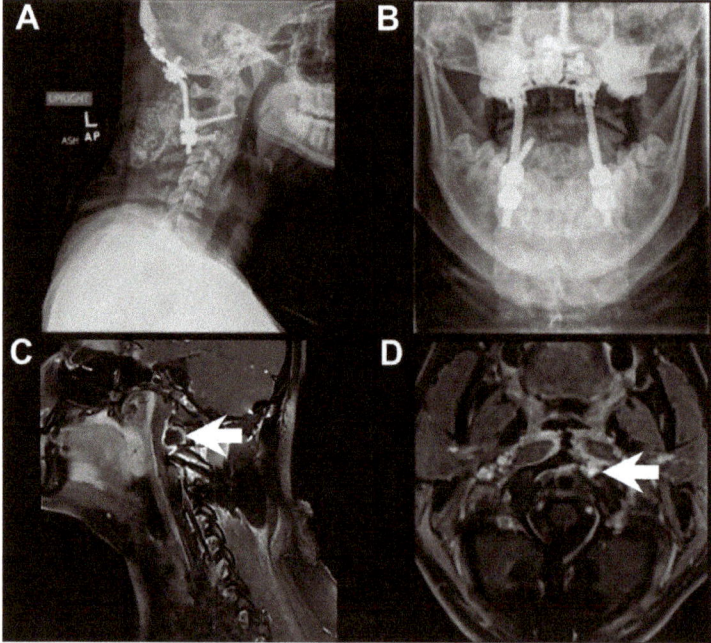

Figure 3. Post-Operative Imaging Studies. Lateral view X-ray of the cervical spine demonstrating hardware on the occiput connected by rods to pedicle screws in C2 and lateral mass screws in C3 bilaterally (**A**). Open mouth odontoid view X-ray demonstrates normal symmetry of C1 and C2 articulation (**B**). Post-contrast MRI T1, sagittal view, demonstrates minimal rim-enhancement within the left lateral C1 representing mild residual tumor (white arrow) (**C**). Post-contrast MRI T1, axial view, of the residual lesion (white arrow) (**D**).

3. Discussion

The differential diagnosis for a spinal column tumor in a pediatric patient is broad, ranging from primary osseous lesions like osteochondromas and osteosarcomas, to tumors of soft tissue origin like rhabdomyosarcoma or neuroblastoma. If the patient's age is taken into consideration, the most common primary osseous tumors in the pediatric spinal column are as follows: 0–5 years of age: eosinophilic granuloma; 5–10 years of age: aneurysmal bone cyst, eosinophilic granuloma, osteoblastoma, osteoid osteoma, osteosarcoma, and Ewing sarcoma; lastly 10–20 years of age: aneurysmal bone cyst, osteochondroma, osteoid osteoma, osteosarcoma, Ewing sarcoma [5].

The most common primary osseous tumor in children is osteochondroma, which makes up about 4% of solitary spinal column tumors. They are benign lesions that consist of an abnormal outgrowth of bone with cartilaginous cap [4]. When these occur in the spine, they occur most often in the cervical spine and must be considered when evaluating a solitary spinal mass in a pediatric patient [6–8]. Of note, about 10% of these tumors will undergo malignant transformation to osteosarcoma. These tumors are usually seen in patients from ages 10–20 and make up about 5% of all spinal lesions [4,9].

The most common malignant primary bone tumor seen in the spinal column of pediatric patients is Ewing sarcoma. Interestingly, these lesions can either arise as primary spinal lesions, or metastasize from other locations to the spine, a characteristic not usually seen in other primary osseous lesions. Ewing sarcoma has a predilection for the sacrum and are found less commonly in the lumbar, thoracic spine, and cervical spine, with decreasing frequency [10]. Osteoblastoma and osteoid osteoma are very pathologically similar primary osseous lesions. They differ mainly in size and behavior, and spinal lesions are most commonly found in the lumbar region [11]. Osteoblastomas are larger, generally greater than 2 cm, and tend to be locally aggressive whereas osteoid osteomas tend to be smaller than 1 cm and more latent, tending to "burn out" over time [12,13].

Another benign primary osseous lesion that can arise in the spine is the aneurysmal bone cyst. These lesions typically present in patients that are 20 years of age or younger and usually affect the lumbar spine [14,15]. Of note, these lesions can invade the pedicles and vertebral bodies on multiple vertebral levels [16]. Lastly, Langerhans cell histiocytosis is a common finding that can be seen in any bone, but occurs in the spine in approximately 10%–15% of cases [5]. The thoracic and cervical spinal regions tend to be the most common locations for this entity [17,18].

Management of most osseous spinal lesions involves en bloc resection with clear margins to avoid tumor recurrence and can be followed by adjuvant therapy, if indicated by pathologic analysis [19,20]. However, careful consideration must be taken to determine the best approach to a spinal column tumor, especially if it is in the cervical region. Tumors in the posterior aspect of the cervical spine usually require a posterior approach with the patient in the prone position [21]. Tumors along the anterior aspect of the spine present a more difficult management dilemma. The anatomy in this region is highly complex and involves many critical neurovascular structures that must be preserved to maintain the patient's post-operative functional status. The transoral approach, which was originally pioneered by Kanavel in 1917, allows for midline access to a wider surgical field with access to multiple cervical vertebrae from C1 to C4 with less compromise to key neurovascular structures [22,23]. This approach has been used in the past to access the anterior cervical spine as noted by Tuite et al. in their report on 27 pediatric patients with occipitocervical junction pathology [24]. They also note that while this approach could have associated morbidity, such as temporomandibular joint dislocation, pharyngeal infection, and swallowing complications, when a standard transoral approach is completed and the hard palate is not compromised, the approach is safe and well tolerated [24,25]. Interestingly, this anatomic region has also been approached via the trans-nasal route as noted by Grammatica et al. This approach is well suited for patients with smaller oral cavities, that would limit the transoral approach and may represent decreased patient morbidity due to the lack of oral retraction during the procedure [26]. However, in cases where tumor pathology is quite lateral in its extent, trans-nasal approach would not allow for proper visualization of key neurovascular structures and would hinder the gross total resection.

To prevent occipitocervical instability, it is often necessary to reconstruct elements of the cervical vertebral column after tumor extirpation. Instability is usually due to a combination of destruction of local anatomy by the tumor and correlates to extent of bony and ligamentous removal during surgery [21]. In these cases, posterior cervical fusion is warranted. In the patient presented here, given extent of bony C1 removal, compromising the ability to place hardware into C1, an occiput to cervical three construct was required for adequate stabilization.

4. Conclusions

Here we report a case of an osteolytic lesion that was incidentally found in the cervical spine of a pediatric patient. The relevant differential diagnosis, as well as surgical techniques involved in treating this patient, have been thoroughly discussed. Anatomy of the atlantooccipital and atlantoaxial joint spaces is complex and medical management of osteolytic lesions discovered in this area should be considered as first-line treatment. However, when the offending lesion is locally aggressive and does not respond to medical management, one must consider surgical intervention for attempted gross total resection, with stabilization of the cranio-vertebral junction. Stabilization of the aforementioned junction using instrumented fusion is key to prevention of patient morbidity and mortality. It is our hope that the information presented will guide surgical decision-making. It is critical to be able to correctly identify the patient population that would most likely benefit from neurosurgical interventions, in the context of rare osteolytic conditions affecting the cervical spine.

Author Contributions: Conceptualization, T.M., C.C.D., C.Z. and A.K.; Methodology, T.M., C.C.D., C.Z. and A.K.; Formal Analysis, T.M., C.C.D., C.Z. and A.K.; Investigation, T.M., C.C.D., C.Z. and A.K.; Resources, T.M., C.C.D., C.Z. and A.K.; Writing—original draft preparation, C.H., V.G., T.M. and C.Z.; Writing—review and editing, C.H., V.G., T.M. and C.Z.; Supervision, T.M. and C.Z.; Project administration, T.M. and C.Z.

Funding: This research received no external funding.

Conflicts of Interest: The authors declare no conflict of interest.

References

1. Rosemberg, S.; Fujiwara, D. Epidemiology of pediatric tumors of the nervous system according to the WHO 2000 classification: A report of 1,195 cases from a single institution. *Child's Nerv. Syst.* **2005**, *21*, 940–944. [CrossRef] [PubMed]
2. Vincent, F.; Fehlings, M.G.; Nater, A. Spinal column tumors. In *Neuro-Concology: The Essentials*; Bernstein, M., Berger, M., Eds.; Thieme: New York, NY, USA, 2000; pp. 391–402.
3. West, R. Childhood cancer mortality: International comparisons 1955–1974. *World Health Stat. Q. Rapp. Trimest. Stat. Sanit. Mond.* **1984**, *37*, 98–127.
4. Harter, D.; Weiner, H. Spinal tumors. In *Principles and Practice of Pediatric Neurosurgery*; Albright, A.L., Pollack, I., Adelson, P., Eds.; Thieme: New York, NY, USA, 2014.
5. Ravindra, V.M.; Eli, I.M.; Schmidt, M.H.; Brockmeyer, D.L. Primary osseous tumors of the pediatric spinal column: Review of pathology and surgical decision making. *Neurosurg. Focus* **2016**, *41*, E3. [CrossRef]
6. Albrecht, S.; Crutchfield, J.S.; SeGall, G.K. On spinal osteochondromas. *J. Neurosurg.* **1992**, *77*, 247–252. [CrossRef]
7. Sharma, M.C.; Arora, R.; Deol, P.S.; Mahapatra, A.K.; Mehta, V.S.; Sarkar, C. Osteochondroma of the spine: An enigmatic tumor of the spinal cord. A series of 10 cases. *J. Neurosurg. Sci.* **2002**, *46*, 66–70; discussion 70. [PubMed]
8. Zaijun, L.; Xinhai, Y.; Zhipeng, W.; Wending, H.; Quan, H.; Zhenhua, Z.; Dapeng, F.; Jisheng, Z.; Wei, Z.; Jianru, X. Outcome and prognosis of myelopathy and radiculopathy from osteochondroma in the mobile spine: A report on 14 patients. *J. Spinal Disord. Technol.* **2013**, *26*, 194–199. [CrossRef]
9. Ilaslan, H.; Sundaram, M.; Unni, K.K.; Shives, T.C. Primary vertebral osteosarcoma: Imaging findings. *Radiology* **2004**, *230*, 697–702. [CrossRef] [PubMed]
10. Venkateswaran, L.; Rodriguez-Galindo, C.; Merchant, T.E.; Poquette, C.A.; Rao, B.N.; Pappo, A.S. Primary Ewing tumor of the vertebrae: Clinical characteristics, prognostic factors, and outcome. *Med. Pediatr. Oncol.* **2001**, *37*, 30–35. [CrossRef] [PubMed]
11. Saifuddin, A.; White, J.; Sherazi, Z.; Shaikh, M.I.; Natali, C.; Ransford, A.O. Osteoid osteoma and osteoblastoma of the spine. Factors associated with the presence of scoliosis. *Spine* **1998**, *23*, 47–53. [CrossRef] [PubMed]
12. Dormans, J.P.; Moroz, L. Infection and tumors of the spine in children. *J. Bone Joint Surg. Am.* **2007**, *89* (Suppl. 1), 79–97.
13. McLeod, R.A.; Dahlin, D.C.; Beabout, J.W. The spectrum of osteoblastoma. *A.J.R. Am. J. Roentgenol.* **1976**, *126*, 321–325. [CrossRef]
14. Hay, M.C.; Paterson, D.; Taylor, T.K. Aneurysmal bone cysts of the spine. *J. Bone Joint Surg. Br.* **1978**, *60*, 406–411. [CrossRef] [PubMed]
15. Lifeso, R.M.; Younge, D. Aneurysmal bone cysts of the spine. *Int. Orthop.* **1985**, *8*, 281–285. [CrossRef] [PubMed]
16. Capanna, R.; Albisinni, U.; Picci, P.; Calderoni, P.; Campanacci, M.; Springfield, D.S. Aneurysmal bone cyst of the spine. *J. Bone Joint Surg. Am.* **1985**, *67*, 527–531. [CrossRef]
17. Greenlee, J.D.W.; Fenoy, A.J.; Donovan, K.A.; Menezes, A.H. Eosinophilic granuloma in the pediatric spine. *Pediatr. Neurosurg.* **2007**, *43*, 285–292. [CrossRef] [PubMed]

18. Levine, S.E.; Dormans, J.P.; Meyer, J.S.; Corcoran, T.A. Langerhans' cell histiocytosis of the spine in children. *Clin. Orthop.* **1996**, 288–293. [CrossRef]
19. Cloyd, J.M.; Acosta, F.L.; Polley, M.-Y.; Ames, C.P. En bloc resection for primary and metastatic tumors of the spine: A systematic review of the literature. *Neurosurgery* **2010**, *67*, 435–444. [CrossRef]
20. Boriani, S.; Bandiera, S.; Biagini, R.; Bacchini, P.; Boriani, L.; Cappuccio, M.; Chevalley, F.; Gasbarrini, A.; Picci, P.; Weinstein, J.N. Chordoma of the mobile spine: Fifty years of experience. *Spine* **2006**, *31*, 493–503. [CrossRef] [PubMed]
21. Jiang, H.; He, J.; Zhan, X.; He, M.; Zong, S.; Xiao, Z. Occipito-cervical fusion following gross total resection for the treatment of spinal extramedullary tumors in craniocervical junction: A retrospective case series. *World J. Surg. Oncol.* **2015**, *13*, 279. [CrossRef] [PubMed]
22. Ortega-Porcayo, L.A.; Cabrera-Aldana, E.E.; Arriada-Mendicoa, N.; Gómez-Amador, J.L.; Granados-García, M.; Barges-Coll, J. Operative technique for en bloc resection of upper cervical chordomas: Extended transoral transmandibular approach and multilevel reconstruction. *Asian Spine J.* **2014**, *8*, 820–826. [PubMed]
23. Kanavel, A.B. Bullet located between the atlas and the base of the skull: Technique of removal through the mouth. *Surg. Clin. Chic.* **1917**, *1*, 361–366.
24. Tuite, G.F.; Veres, R.; Crockard, H.A.; Sell, D. Pediatric transoral surgery: Indications, complications, and long-term outcome. *J. Neurosurg.* **1996**, *84*, 573–583. [CrossRef]
25. Salem, K.M.I.; Visser, J.; Quraishi, N.A. Trans-oral approach for the management of a C2 neuroblastoma. *Eur. Spine J.* **2015**, *24*, 170–176. [CrossRef]
26. Grammatica, A.; Bonali, M.; Ruscitti, F.; Marchioni, D.; Pinna, G.; Cunsolo, E.M.; Presutti, L. Transnasal endoscopic removal of malformation of the odontoid process in a patient with type I Arnold-Chiari malformation: A case report. *Acta Otorhinolaryngol. Ital.* **2011**, *31*, 248–252.

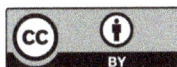

© 2019 by the authors. Licensee MDPI, Basel, Switzerland. This article is an open access article distributed under the terms and conditions of the Creative Commons Attribution (CC BY) license (http://creativecommons.org/licenses/by/4.0/).

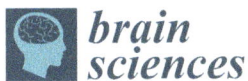

Case Report

Endogenous Neurostimulation and Physiotherapy in Cluster Headache: A Clinical Case

Gonzalo Navarro-Fernández [1,2], Lucía de-la-Puente-Ranea [1], Marisa Gandía-González [3] and Alfonso Gil-Martínez [1,2,4,*]

1. Departamento de Fisioterapia, Centro Superior de Estudios Universitarios La Salle, Universidad Autónoma de Madrid, Madrid 28023, Spain; gonza_navarro93@hotmail.com (G.N.-F.); luciadelapuenteranea@gmail.com (L.d.-l.-P.-R.)
2. Motion in Brains Research Group, Instituto de Neurociencias y Ciencias del Movimiento, Centro Superior de Estudios Universitarios La Salle, Universidad Autónoma de Madrid, Madrid 28023, Spain
3. Servicio de Neurocirugía, Hospital Universitario La Paz, Madrid 28046, Spain; marisagg4@hotmail.com
4. Hospital La Paz Institute for Health Research, Madrid 28046, Spain
* Correspondence: fongilmar@gmail.com

Received: 15 February 2019; Accepted: 8 March 2019; Published: 12 March 2019

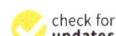

Abstract: Objective: The aim of this paper is to describe the progressive changes of chronic cluster headaches (CHs) in a patient who is being treated by a multimodal approach, using pharmacology, neurostimulation and physiotherapy. Subject: A male patient, 42 years of age was diagnosed with left-sided refractory chronic CH by a neurologist in November 2009. In June 2014, the patient underwent a surgical intervention in which a bilateral occipital nerve neurostimulator was implanted as a treatment for headache. Methods: Case report. Results: Primary findings included a decreased frequency of CH which lasted up to 2 months and sometimes even without pain. Besides this, there were decreased levels of anxiety, helplessness (PCS subscale) and a decreased impact of headache (HIT-6 scale). Bilateral pressure pain thresholds (PPTs) were improved along with an increase in strength and motor control of the neck muscles. These improvements were present at the conclusion of the treatment and maintained up to 4 months after the treatment. Conclusions: A multimodal approach, including pharmacology, neurostimulation and physiotherapy may be beneficial for patients with chronic CHs. Further studies such as case series and clinical trials are needed to confirm these results.

Keywords: cluster headache; neurosurgery; pressure pain threshold; physiotherapy

1. Introduction

The cluster headache (CH) has been defined by the International Headache Society as the most frequent trigeminal autonomic headache [1]. CHs is reported to be found in 0.12% of the population, with an overall male-to-female ratio of 3:1; episodic CH is more common than chronic CH [2,3]. CHs are characterized by severe unilateral pain in short-duration episodes, which are associated with ipsilateral autonomic symptoms which primarily encompass the temporal, supraorbital and infraorbital areas [1,3].

Much research performed in the early 2000s confirmed the involvement of the changes in the hypothalamus in patients with CH. For instance, May et al. concluded that there were activation and structural changes in the gray matter of the posterior and inferior parts of the hypothalamus [4]. More recent studies have also shown that there is hypothalamus activation in patients with CH, but there are no structural changes in the gray matter in that area, unlike other regions in which morphological changes were found, such as the hippocampus, anterior insula, orbitofrontal cortex, cerebellum, temporal lobe, anterior cingulate cortex and the primary and secondary somatosensory cortex [5]. The convergence theory describes the anatomo-functional convergence of the cervical (especially C2), somatic trigeminal and dural trigeminovascular afferent neurons on second-order nociceptors in the trigeminocervical complex [6]. One of the supporting studies found limited duration, frequency and intensity of cluster attacks after blockades, asserting the theory of convergence [7–9].

These findings could, therefore, be related to the extensive effect of pharmacological treatments proposed for patients with CH, such as sumatriptan, [3,10,11] other triptans, [12,13] verapamil, [13] lithium, [3,13] oxygen therapy, [14] onabotulinumtoxinA [15] and alternative treatments such as valproic acid, topiramate and methylprednisone [13].

The American Headache Society only proposes pharmacological and oxygen therapy as acute treatment with "A" level recommendation [16]. The lack of evidence makes the inclusion of other therapies in the evidence-based treatment guidelines more difficult. Moreover, the review of the effects of the principal drugs used in the treatment of acute CH shows side effects such as chest pain, paresthesia, dizziness, tingling feeling or numbness of the limbs, heaviness, asthenia, nausea, unpleasant taste, and somnolence [17,18]. Somatostatin treatment also has some side effects, and the most frequent among them are hyperglycaemia, nausea, abdomianal pain, diarrhea, and meteorism [18]. Adverse effects are also present in prophylactic treatments. Lithium carbonate produces tremor, gastrointestinal disturbances, dizziness, olfactory disorders and polyuria in CH patients [18–20]. Even though verapamil has been considered as the first-line prophylactic drug for the treatment of CH patients with "A" level recommendation [13], it should be used carefully, because verapramil treatment is noted to have a correlation with the electrocardiographic abnormalities (19% arrhythmias and 36% of bradycardia incidence) [21].

Limitations of drug treatment are advised in both episodic and chronic CH because 10% to 20% of CCHs have the chance of becoming drug-resistant headaches [22], and a new line in the research has been opened to increase the use of non-pharmacological adjuvant treatments for CH.

There are some non-invasive stimulation methods that have been used in CH patients. At first, the results obtained by Nesbitt et al. in 2015 suggested that non-invasive vagal nerve stimulation can be used as both acute and prophylactic treatment in ECH and CCH [23]. However, it has recently been shown that non-invasive vagal nerve stimulation is an effective treatment in ECH when compared with sham stimulation, but not in the CCH patient group [24]. Additionally, some investigators are assessing the effects obtained by using transcranial magnetic stimulation techniques in CH [25,26], but the evidence is still limited [27].

One of the most investigated invasive stimulation methods is sphenopalatine ganglion stimulation (SPG). This method was used in a study published in 2017, and it was concluded that after 24 months, 45% of the patients with refractory CCH were acute responders and 35% were frequent responders. Even though 81% of the side effect incidences were reported, they noted that SPG produced 61% of therapeutic responses and should be considered as an interesting treatment for refractory CCH [28]. Another invasive stimulation method commonly used in CH patients is occipital nerve stimulation (ONS). Although it has shown that ONS can reduce the frequency and intensity of headache at least by a 50% in about 60% of the patients [29], there is a lack of randomized controlled trials of ONS for the treatment of CH [27].

Moreover, manual therapies are being investigated in other primary headache cases; studies have shown that manual therapy was significantly better in the control group in reducing the intensity and frequency of headache [30].

Our aim was to describe the management of chronic CH in a patient who is treated by a multimodal approach including pharmacology, neurostimulation and physiotherapy.

2. Methods

The CARE (case reporting guideline development) checklist was used to prepare this case report and to complete it to improve quality reports in clinical cases [31].

2.1. Patient

A male patient of 42 years of age was diagnosed with left-sided refractory chronic CH by a neurologist in November 2009. The following pharmacological treatment was prescribed by the neurologist: (1) preventive treatment: verapamil (80 mg), topiramate (100 mg), escitalopram (15 mg), clonazepam (0.5 mg), lithium (100 mg) and prednisone (25 mg); and (2) abortive treatment: subcutaneous sumatriptan injection (6 mg) and 100% oxygen. The patient reported loss of memory and concentration as an adverse effect of the medication. In June 2014, the patient underwent a surgical intervention in which a bilateral occipital nerve neurostimulator was implanted as the treatment method for headache.

2.2. Neurostimulator Implantation Procedure

To establish a subcutaneous stimulation of the greater occipital nerve complex, the implantation of bilateral 8-contact occipital lead was performed, using anatomical and radiological landmarks.

Surgery was performed with the patient lying in the prone position and completely awake. Under local anesthesia, a midline incision in the back of the neck was made with a small epifascial scalpel. Guided by an anteroposterior X-ray image, a subcutaneous needle followed the curvature of the skin from the C1–C2 transition to the mastoid process on one side, avoiding the perforation of the fascia to prevent subfascial electrode localization on the other side.

The electrodes were placed subcutaneously and the needles were removed. The electrodes were anchored in the fascia after checking the correct coverage of the target area, and then two loops were placed. The electrodes were tunneled to the subcutaneous point at the halfway point between the midline neck incision and the subcutaneous gluteal buttock (on the right or left side, depending on the patient's preference), where the another set of loops lay, which were attached to each electrode and then connected with the extensions (Figure 1). To identified the greater occipital nerve complex correctly, some serial ultrasound images and videos published by Chang KV et al. were used [32].

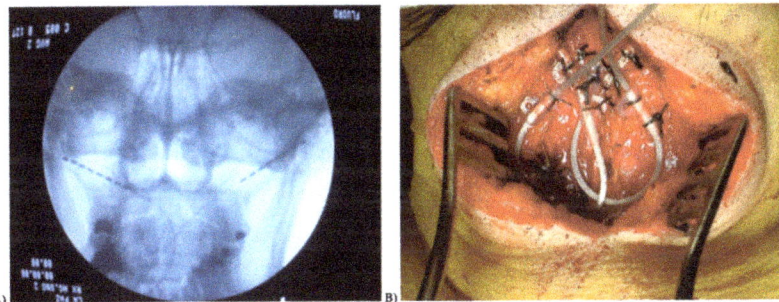

Figure 1. (**A**) Anteroposterior X-ray electrode image, after removing the needles, prepared for stimulation; (**B**) fascia anchor in suboccipital level.

The extensions were tunneled to the subcutaneous gluteal buttock, where the implantable pulse generator was definitively placed after the extensions were connected and the correct impedances and stimulation were verified. Incision closure was performed when the correct hemostasis had occurred.

2.3. Evaluation

After signing the informed consent, the patient was evaluated before the treatment procedure, after the treatment, and at the 3rd month and 4th month after the treatment. A blinded experienced evaluator assessed both physical and psychological variables, which were selected according to previous observational studies in patients with CH [33]. Physical variables were pressure pain thresholds (PPTs) assessed bilaterally in the cranial and extracranial areas with a digital algometer [34]

(Fx. 25 Force Gage, Wagner Instruments, Greenwich, CT, USA); two-point discrimination was tested in the trigeminal areas with an esthesiometer [35]; and cervical flexor endurance was measured with a craniocervical flexion test [36]. Psychological variables were as follows: impact of headache on the quality of life and work performance (HIT-6 scale) [37], pain catastrophizing (PC Scale) [38], neck disability (neck disability Index) [39] and depression symptoms (Hamilton depression rating scale) [40]. At each assessment, we measured the impact and outcome of disease in the patient's daily life (with a verbal numeric rating scale) [41], the intensity and frequency of pain, crisis duration and medication used in each episode, and all the data were recorded in a diary.

After observing the values obtained in the first assessment session, such as the reduced endurance of deep flexor cervical muscles (Table 1), the authors decided to include physical therapy as an adjuvant treatment for the patients.

Table 1. Data and % of change of physical variables and psychological characteristics.

	Pre	Post	3 Months	4 Months	% of Change
PPT					% Pre-4 months
V1 right	1.12	0.75	1.71	1.49	33.03%
V2 right	1.62	1.22	2.45	2.77	70.98%
V3 right	1.39	0.94	2.5	1.67	20.14%
Temporalis M1 right	2.58	2.13	4.17	2.73	5.81%
Temporalis M2 right	3.28	3.19	5.7	5.16	57.32%
V1 left	0.72	0.62	1.52	1.29	79.17%
V2 left	1.27	1.08	2.86	3.1	144.09%
V3 left	1.37	0.88	3.03	2.41	75.91%
Temporalis M1 left	1.69	2.09	3.28	3.56	110.65%
Temporalis M2 left	2.85	3.19	5.35	4.64	62.81%
Mastoid P right	3.54	3.34	4.54	4.64	31.07%
Mastoid P left	2.81	2.14	3.52	4.2	49.47%
Greater occipital N right	4.75	3.8	4.68	4.04	−14.95%
Greater occipital N left	4.34	3.26	4.64	3.42	−21.20%
Tibialis M right	4.98	6.31	17.6	10.96	120.08%
Tibialis M left	5.84	5.17	17.08	12.68	117.12%
Craniocervical flexion test time (s)	3.06	8.22	12.47	24.06	-
Fatigue	21.5	22	43	60.5	-
Physiological characteristic differences Pre-4 months					
HIT-6	63	61	50	54	−9
NDI	18	12	13	13	−5
PCS	17	10	10	10	−7
PCS rumination	8	7	7	7	−1
PCS magnification	0	0	0	0	0
PCS helplessness	9	3	3	3	−6
HDRS	20	18	14	14	−6

PPT = pressure pain threshold; M = muscle; N = nerve; P = process; HIT-6 = headache impact test; NDI = neck disability index; PCS = pain catastrophizing scale; HDRS = Hamilton depression rating scale.

2.4. Postsurgical Physiotherapy Approach

The patient received 8 physical therapy sessions in 6 weeks. Manual therapy techniques consisted of passive mobilization of the anterior–posterior upper cervical region, which can directly influence the upper three cervical segments (C0–C3), and three sets of 2 minutes of mobilization were performed with 0.5 Hz frequency and 30 seconds of rest [42]; additionally, the neurodynamic mobilization of the trigeminal nerve was performed, with 30 repetitions with 0.5Hz frequency (10 global mobilizations of mandibular opening and 10 mobilizations on each side of the mandibular laterotrusion to ease the tension to the auriculotemporal nerve) (Figure 2A,B). Finally, home exercises were prescribed to improve the motor control of deep flexor muscles, as described by Harris et al., [43], and the patient was advised to perform three sets of 10–20 repetitions including 5–10 seconds of contraction with 5–10 seconds of relaxation, depending on the patient's strength.

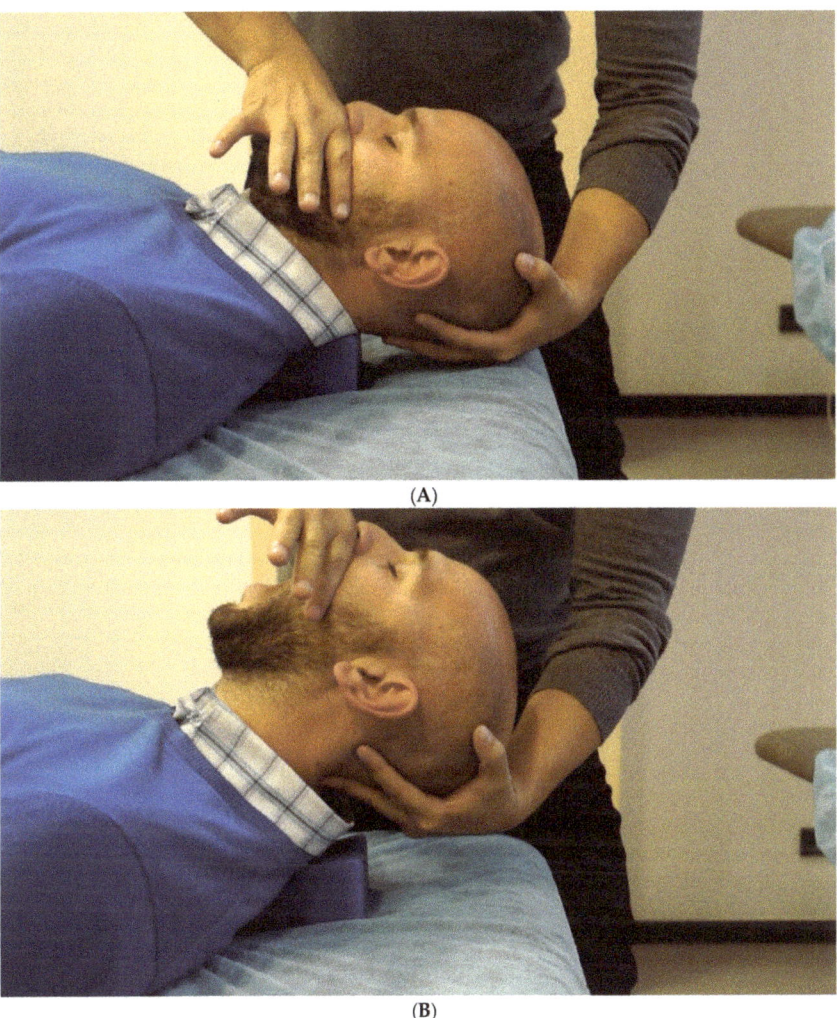

Figure 2. (**A**) Neural mobilization (step 1). Craniocervical flexion; (**B**) neural mobilization (step 2). Craniocervical extension plus mouth opening.

3. Results and Discussion

This is the first case to be reported to receive treatment as a combination of neurostimulation and physiotherapy approaches for chronic CH. After analyzing the patient's case diary of headache, a decreased frequency of CH attacks was observed at the end of treatment, and the progress was maintained even 4 months after the treatment; additionally, it was reported that for the first 2 months there was no pain at all (Table 2). These results could support the use of a multimodal approach as an adjunctive treatment for occipital nerve neurostimulation (C2–C3). The benefits obtained with neurostimulation treatment might support the trigeminal–cervical convergence hypothesis [44,45], according to which craniofacial pain is generated by the activation of second-order neurons from the trigeminal nucleus caudalis, [45] a mechanism generated both in animals and in humans. [46] Other authors have developed studies in which it was observed that stimulation of the superior sagittal sinus, innervated by the ophthalmic branch of the trigeminus, also take part in the stimulation of second-order neurons of the trigeminal nucleus caudalis and the dorsal horn of C2–C3. Thus, this supports the trigeminal–cervical convergence hypothesis and provides the basis for neurostimulation.

Table 2. Evolution of headache diary.

Months	Frequency	Intensity	Duration	Abortive Treatment
May	2	9	25	SS-OT
June	3	9.33	23.33	SS
July	7	9.71	31.43	SS-OT
August	2	9.50	35	SS
September	0	-	-	-
October	0	-	-	-
November	4	8.50	33.75	SS-OT

SS = subcutaneous sumaptriptan; OT = oxygen therapy.

In addition, physical therapy techniques such as manual therapy, therapeutic exercise or a combination of both, specifically applied in the upper cervical region, had already caused a decrease in the frequency and intensity of various primary headaches. [47–49] These results reinforce our hypothesis that the combination of these techniques might reduce headache frequency due to the activation or inhibition of sensory input from the trigeminal–cervical system [46] in chronic CH.

The decrease in frequency of attacks after the multimodal program can lead to decreased levels of anxiety, helplessness (PCS subscale) and impact of headache (Table 1). Ruscheweyh et al. demonstrated that the frequency of a primary headache is associated with pain-specific disability, quality of life, anxiety and depression, which are significantly more pronounced in patients with a chronic headache than in patients who have episodic attacks [50].

Moreover, the patient showed an improvement (increase) in most PPTs bilaterally, except in those that were examined and assessed on the greater occipital nerve (Table 1). These results could be due to the analgesic effect generated by the joint mobilization [42,51] or trigeminal neural mobilization, [52] along with the pharmacological and neurostimulation treatments. However, the decrease in the occipital nerve PPT coincides with the area of neurostimulator implantation, where the patient had reported a feeling of numbness (paresthesia) [44] that increased while performing a passive lateral glide of C0–C1, which suggests that active and passive craniocervical flexion could generate allodynia at these points, as occurs in CH conditions [53].

Finally, the inclusion of a therapeutic exercise program could also cause an increase in the strength and motor control of the cervical muscle, which was proved by comparing the pretreatment assessment and the assessment at the fourth month after the treatment (Table 1), which is supported by the evidence of the fact that stabilization exercise is effective in reducing pain [54] and might be useful in the treatment of other primary headaches as well [55]. Instead of longer follow-up, it is better to make the patient aware of the fact that the combination of neurostimulation and physiotherapy could be effective in reducing the frequency, duration, and severity of the CH. This may remove their lack of adherence to the treatment.

Finally, the limitation should be marked that, currently, ultrasound is widely used in assessing neuromuscular disorders. Some headaches could result from the chronic affection of the para-spinal and sub-occipital muscles, which can be easily checked by using ultrasound [32]. Unfortunately, the authors did not use this to examine possible musculoskeletal painful origins in this single case.

In conclusion, a multimodal approach, including pharmacology, neurostimulation and physiotherapy, could be beneficial in the management of patients with chronic CH.

Author Contributions: Conceptualization, G.N.-F., L.d.-l.-P.-R. and A.G.-M.; methodology, A.G.-M.; software, A.G.-M.; formal analysis, G.N.-F., L.d.-l.-P.-R. and A.G.-M.; investigation, G.N.-F., L.d.-l.-P.-R., M.G.-G. and A.G.-M.; resources, G.N.-F. and L.d.-l.-P.-R.; data curation, G.N.-F. and L.d.-l.-P.-R.; writing—original draft preparation, G.N.-F. and L.d.-l.-P.-R.; writing—review and editing, M.G.-G. and A.G.-M.; visualization, A.G.-M.; supervision, A.G.-M.; project administration, A.G.-M.

Funding: This research received no external funding.

Conflicts of Interest: The authors declare no conflict of interest.

Clinical Implications: Most of the current treatments available for patients with a cluster headache are unsatisfactory. This is the first study that reports the benefits of a multimodal approach, which could be a promising line of research for this complex problem of patients. Further studies, such as case series and clinical trials, are needed to confirm these results.

References

1. Headache Classification Committee of the International Headache Society (IHS). The International Classification of Headache Disorders, 3rd edition (beta version). *Cephalalgia* **2013**, *33*, 629–808. [CrossRef]
2. Fischera, M.; Marziniak, M.; Gralow, I.; Evers, S. The incidence and prevalence of cluster headache: A meta-analysis of population-based studies. *Cephalalgia* **2008**, *28*, 614–618. [CrossRef]
3. Meyers, S.L. Cluster headache and trigeminal autonomic cephalgias. *Dis. Mon.* **2015**, *61*, 236–239. [CrossRef]
4. May, A.; Bahra, A.; Büchel, C.; Frackowiak, R.S.; Goadsby, P.J. PET and MRA findings in cluster headache and MRA in experimental pain. *Neurology* **2000**, *55*, 1328–1335. [CrossRef]
5. Naegel, S.; Holle, D.; Desmarattes, N.; Theysohn, N.; Diener, H.-C.; Katsarava, Z.; Obermann, M. Cortical plasticity in episodic and chronic cluster headache. *Neuroimage Clin.* **2014**, *6*, 415–423. [CrossRef] [PubMed]
6. Bartsch, T.; Goadsby, P.J. Stimulation of the greater occipital nerve induces increased central excitability of dural afferent input. *Brain* **2002**, *125*, 1496–1509. [CrossRef] [PubMed]
7. Afridi, S.K.; Shields, K.G.; Bhola, R.; Goadsby, P.J. Greater occipital nerve injection in primary headache syndromes–prolonged effects from a single injection. *Pain* **2006**, *122*, 126–129. [CrossRef] [PubMed]
8. Ambrosini, A.; Vandenheede, M.; Rossi, P.; Aloj, F.; Sauli, E.; Pierelli, F.; Schoenen, J. Suboccipital injection with a mixture of rapid- and long-acting steroids in cluster headache: A double-blind placebo-controlled study. *Pain* **2005**, *118*, 92–96. [CrossRef] [PubMed]
9. Peres, M.F.P.; Stiles, M.A.; Siow, H.C.; Rozen, T.D.; Young, W.B.; Silberstein, S.D. Greater occipital nerve blockade for cluster headache. *Cephalalgia* **2002**, *22*, 520–522. [CrossRef]
10. Leone, M.; Proietti Cecchini, A. Long-term use of daily sumatriptan injections in severe drug-resistant chronic cluster headache. *Neurology* **2015**, *86*, 194–195. [CrossRef]
11. Ekbom, K.; Monstad, I.; Prusinski, A.; Cole, J.A.; Pilgrim, A.J.; Noronha, D. Subcutaneous sumatriptan in the acute treatment of cluster headache: A dose comparison study. The Sumatriptan Cluster Headache Study Group. *Acta Neurol. Scand.* **1993**, *88*, 63–69. [CrossRef] [PubMed]
12. Law, S.; Derry, S.; Moore, R.A. Triptans for acute cluster headache. *Cochrane Database Syst. Rev.* **2013**, *7*, CD008042. [CrossRef] [PubMed]
13. May, A.; Leone, M.; Afra, J.; Linde, M.; Sándor, P.S.; Evers, S.; Goadsby, P.J. EFNS guidelines on the treatment of cluster headache and other trigeminal-autonomic cephalalgias. *Eur. J. Neurol.* **2006**, *13*, 1066–1077. [CrossRef] [PubMed]
14. Petersen, A.S.; Barloese, M.C.; Jensen, R.H. Oxygen treatment of cluster headache: A review. *Cephalalgia* **2014**, *34*, 1079–1087. [CrossRef]
15. Bratbak, D.F.; Nordgård, S.; Stovner, L.J.; Linde, M.; Folvik, M.; Bugten, V.; Tronvik, E. Pilot study of sphenopalatine injection of onabotulinumtoxinA for the treatment of intractable chronic cluster headache. *Cephalalgia* **2015**, *36*, 503–509. [CrossRef] [PubMed]
16. Robbins, M.S.; Starling, A.J.; Pringsheim, T.M.; Becker, W.J.; Schwedt, T.J. Treatment of Cluster Headache: The American Headache Society Evidence-Based Guidelines. *Headache J. Head Face Pain* **2016**, *56*, 1093–1106. [CrossRef] [PubMed]
17. Gregor, N.; Schlesiger, C.; Akova-Ozturk, E.; Kraemer, C.; Husstedt, I.-W.; Evers, S. Treatment of Cluster Headache Attacks With Less Than 6 mg Subcutaneous Sumatriptan. *Headache J. Head Face Pain* **2005**, *45*, 1069–1072. [CrossRef] [PubMed]

18. Costa, A.; Antonaci, F.; Ramusino, M.C.; Nappi, G. The Neuropharmacology of Cluster Headache and other Trigeminal Autonomic Cephalalgias. *Curr. Neuropharmacol.* **2015**, *13*, 304–323. [CrossRef]
19. Savoldi, F.; Bono, G.; Manzoni, G.C.; Micieli, G.; Lanfranchi, M.; Nappi, G. Lithium salts in cluster headache treatment. *Cephalalgia* **1983**, *3*, 79–84. [CrossRef] [PubMed]
20. Bussone, G.; Leone, M.; Peccarisi, C.; Micieli, G.; Granella, F.; Magri, M.; Manzoni, G.C.; Nappi, G. Double blind comparison of lithium and verapamil in cluster headache prophylaxis. *Headache* **1990**, *30*, 411–417. [CrossRef]
21. Cohen, A.S.; Matharu, M.S.; Goadsby, P.J. Electrocardiographic abnormalities in patients with cluster headache on verapamil therapy. *Neurology* **2007**, *69*, 668–675. [CrossRef]
22. Leone, M.; Franzini, A.; Proietti Cecchini, A.; Mea, E.; Broggi, G.; Bussone, G. Costs of hypothalamic stimulation in chronic drug-resistant cluster headache: Preliminary data. *Neurol. Sci.* **2009**, *30*, 43–47. [CrossRef]
23. Nesbitt, A.D.; Marin, J.C.A.; Tompkins, E.; Ruttledge, M.H.; Goadsby, P.J. Initial use of a novel noninvasive vagus nerve stimulator for cluster headache treatment. *Neurology* **2015**, *84*, 1249–1253. [CrossRef]
24. Goadsby, P.J.; de Coo, I.F.; Silver, N.; Tyagi, A.; Ahmed, F.; Gaul, C.; Jensen, R.H.; Diener, H.-C.; Solbach, K.; Straube, A.; et al. Non-invasive vagus nerve stimulation for the acute treatment of episodic and chronic cluster headache: A randomized, double-blind, sham-controlled ACT2 study. *Cephalalgia* **2017**, *38*, 959–969. [CrossRef]
25. Cosentino, G.; Brighina, F.; Brancato, S.; Valentino, F.; Indovino, S.; Fierro, B. Transcranial magnetic stimulation reveals cortical hyperexcitability in episodic cluster headache. *J. Pain* **2015**, *16*, 53–59. [CrossRef]
26. Hodaj, H.; Alibeu, J.-P.; Payen, J.-F.; Lefaucheur, J.-P. Treatment of Chronic Facial Pain Including Cluster Headache by Repetitive Transcranial Magnetic Stimulation of the Motor Cortex with Maintenance Sessions: A Naturalistic Study. *Brain Stimul.* **2015**, *8*, 801–807. [CrossRef]
27. Schwedt, T.J.; Vargas, B. Neurostimulation for Treatment of Migraine and Cluster Headache. *Pain Med.* **2015**, *16*, 1827–1834. [CrossRef]
28. Jürgens, T.P.; Barloese, M.; May, A.; Láinez, J.M.; Schoenen, J.; Gaul, C.; Goodman, A.M.; Caparso, A.; Jensen, R.H. Long-term effectiveness of sphenopalatine ganglion stimulation for cluster headache. *Cephalalgia* **2017**, *37*, 423–434. [CrossRef]
29. Magis, D.; Schoenen, J. Advances and challenges in neurostimulation for headaches. *Lancet. Neurol.* **2012**, *11*, 708–719. [CrossRef]
30. Chaibi, A.; Russell, M.B. Manual therapies for cervicogenic headache: A systematic review. *J. Headache Pain* **2012**, *13*, 351–359. [CrossRef]
31. Gagnier, J.J.; Kienle, G.; Altman, D.G.; Moher, D.; Sox, H.; Riley, D. CARE Group the CARE guidelines: Consensus-based clinical case report guideline development. *J. Clin. Epidemiol.* **2014**, *67*, 46–51. [CrossRef] [PubMed]
32. Chang, K.-V.; Lin, C.-P.; Hung, C.-Y.; Özçakar, L.; Wang, T.-G.; Chen, W.-S. Sonographic Nerve Tracking in the Cervical Region: A Pictorial Essay and Video Demonstration. *Am. J. Phys. Med. Rehabil.* **2016**, *95*, 862–870. [CrossRef]
33. Fernández-de-las-Peñas, C.; Ortega-Santiago, R.; Cuadrado, M.L.; López-de-Silanes, C.; Pareja, J.A. Bilateral Widespread Mechanical Pain Hypersensitivity as Sign of Central Sensitization in Patients with Cluster Headache. *Headache J. Head Face Pain* **2011**, *51*, 384–391. [CrossRef]
34. Kinser, A.M.; Sands, W.A.; Stone, M.H. Reliability and validity of a pressure algometer. *J. Strength Cond. Res.* **2009**, *23*, 312–314. [CrossRef] [PubMed]
35. Bulut, T.; Akgun, U.; Ozcan, C.; Unver, B.; Sener, M. Inter- and intra-tester reliability of sensibility testing in digital nerve repair. *J. Hand Surg. Eur.* **2015**, *41*, 621–623. [CrossRef]
36. Olson, L.E.; Millar, A.L.; Dunker, J.; Hicks, J.; Glanz, D. Reliability of a clinical test for deep cervical flexor endurance. *J. Manip. Physiol. Ther.* **2006**, *29*, 134–138. [CrossRef]
37. Sauro, K.M.; Rose, M.S.; Becker, W.J.; Christie, S.N.; Giammarco, R.; Mackie, G.F.; Eloff, A.G.; Gawel, M.J. HIT-6 and MIDAS as measures of headache disability in a headache referral population. *Headache* **2010**, *50*, 383–395. [CrossRef] [PubMed]
38. Olmedilla Zafra, A.; Ortega Toro, E.; Cano, L.A. Validation of the Pain Catastrophizing Scale in Spanish athletes. *Cuadernos Psicologia Deporte* **2013**, *13*, 83–93. [CrossRef]

39. Andrade Ortega, J.A.; Delgado Martínez, A.D.; Almécija Ruiz, R. Validation of the Spanish version of the Neck Disability Index. *Spine* **2010**, *35*, E114–E118. [CrossRef] [PubMed]
40. Lobo, A.; Chamorro, L.; Luque, A.; Dal-Ré, R.; Badia, X.; Baró, E. Validation of the Spanish versions of the Montgomery-Asberg depression and Hamilton anxiety rating scales. *Med. Clin.* **2002**, *118*, 493–499. [CrossRef]
41. Holdgate, A.; Asha, S.; Craig, J.; Thompson, J. Comparison of a verbal numeric rating scale with the visual analogue scale for the measurement of acute pain. *Emerg. Med.* **2003**, *15*, 441–446. [CrossRef]
42. La Touche, R.; París-Alemany, A.; Mannheimer, J.S.; Angulo-Díaz-Parreño, S.; Bishop, M.D.; Lopéz-Valverde-Centeno, A.; von Piekartz, H.; Fernández-Carnero, J. Does mobilization of the upper cervical spine affect pain sensitivity and autonomic nervous system function in patients with cervico-craniofacial pain?: A randomized-controlled trial. *Clin. J. Pain* **2013**, *29*, 205–215. [CrossRef]
43. Harris, K.D.; Heer, D.M.; Roy, T.C.; Santos, D.M.; Whitman, J.M.; Wainner, R.S. Reliability of a measurement of neck flexor muscle endurance. *Phys Ther.* **2005**, *85*, 1349–1355.
44. Rodrigo, M.D.; Quero, J.; Cía, P.; Escartín, R.; Acín, P.; Bono, C.; Polo, C. Estimulación eléctrica invasiva de C2-C3 en el tratamiento del dolor cefálico y facial: Neuralgia occipital. Migraña transformada. Cefalea en racimos. Algias faciales. *Rev. De La Soc. Española Del Dolor* **2008**, *15*, 382–391.
45. Pedersen, J.L.; Barloese, M.; Jensen, R.H. Neurostimulation in cluster headache: A review of current progress. *Cephalalgia* **2013**, *33*, 1179–1193. [CrossRef]
46. Piovesan, E.J.; Kowacs, P.A.; Tatsui, C.E.; Lange, M.C.; Ribas, L.C.; Werneck, L.C. Referred pain after painful stimulation of the greater occipital nerve in humans: Evidence of convergence of cervical afferences on trigeminal nuclei. *Cephalalgia* **2001**, *21*, 107–109. [CrossRef]
47. Busch, V.; Gaul, C. Exercise in migraine therapy is there any evidence for efficacy? A critical review. *Headache* **2008**, *48*, 890–899. [CrossRef]
48. Hall, T.; Chan, H.T.; Christensen, L.; Odenthal, B.; Wells, C.; Robinson, K. Efficacy of a C1-C2 self-sustained natural apophyseal glide (SNAG) in the management of cervicogenic headache. *J. Orthop. Sports Phys. Ther.* **2007**, *37*, 100–107. [CrossRef]
49. Skyba, D.A.; Radhakrishnan, R.; Rohlwing, J.J.; Wright, A.; Sluka, K.A. Joint manipulation reduces hyperalgesia by activation of monoamine receptors but not opioid or GABA receptors in the spinal cord. *Pain* **2003**, *106*, 159–168. [CrossRef]
50. Ruscheweyh, R.; Müller, M.; Blum, B.; Straube, A. Correlation of headache frequency and psychosocial impairment in migraine: A cross-sectional study. *Headache* **2014**, *54*, 861–871. [CrossRef]
51. Chaibi, A.; Russell, M.B. Manual therapies for primary chronic headaches: A systematic review of randomized controlled trials. *J. Headache Pain* **2014**, *15*, 67. [CrossRef]
52. Santos, F.M.; Silva, J.T.; Giardini, A.C.; Rocha, P.A.; Achermann, A.P.P.; Alves, A.S.; Britto, L.R.G.; Chacur, M. Neural mobilization reverses behavioral and cellular changes that characterize neuropathic pain in rats. *Mol. Pain* **2012**, *8*, 57. [CrossRef] [PubMed]
53. Wilbrink, L.A.; Louter, M.A.; Teernstra, O.P.M.; van Zwet, E.W.; Huygen, F.J.P.M.; Haan, J.; Ferrari, M.D.; Terwindt, G.M. Allodynia in cluster headache. *Pain* **2017**, *158*, 1113–1117. [CrossRef]
54. Ferreira, P.H.; Ferreira, M.L.; Maher, C.G.; Herbert, R.D.; Refshauge, K. Specific stabilisation exercise for spinal and pelvic pain: A systematic review. *Aust. J. Physiother.* **2006**, *52*, 79–88. [CrossRef]
55. Gil-Martínez, A.; Kindelan-Calvo, P.; Agudo-Carmona, D.; Muñoz-Plata, R.; López-de-Uralde-Villanueva, I.; La Touche, R. Therapeutic exercise as treatment for migraine and tension-type headaches: A systematic review of randomised clinical trials. *Rev. Neurol.* **2013**, *57*, 433–443.

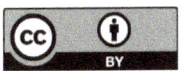

© 2019 by the authors. Licensee MDPI, Basel, Switzerland. This article is an open access article distributed under the terms and conditions of the Creative Commons Attribution (CC BY) license (http://creativecommons.org/licenses/by/4.0/).

MDPI\
St. Alban-Anlage 66\
4052 Basel\
Switzerland\
Tel. +41 61 683 77 34\
Fax +41 61 302 89 18\
www.mdpi.com

Brain Sciences Editorial Office\
E-mail: brainsci@mdpi.com\
www.mdpi.com/journal/brainsci

www.ingramcontent.com/pod-product-compliance
Lightning Source LLC
LaVergne TN
LVHW071444100526
838202LV00088B/6808